PENGUIN BOOKS
DR CUTERUS

DR TANAYA NARENDRA is an internationally trained medical doctor, embryologist, and scientist, who is passionate about medical education.

After studying for a masters at the University of Oxford, she subsequently registered as a doctor in England, and committed to making public medical education her life's goal. She is an elected Fellow of the prestigious Royal Society for Public Health.

For her groundbreaking work in medical education, Tanaya has been awarded Sexual Health Influencer of the Year 2020 by SH24—the online sexual health partner of the NHS; she was also named among the Top 25 Disruptors of India 2021 by *Cosmopolitan*, and was selected the Health Influencer of the Year by the IHW Council, supported by the NITI Aayog and Ayushman Bharat.

She is now the most popular medical professional on social media in India. Tanaya runs @Dr_Cuterus, which has garnered over one million followers on Instagram and over 50 million views on YouTube. She uses fairy tales, mannequins, fun GIFs, and hilariously relatable examples to talk in a jargon-free and scientific manner about complex medical and sexual education topics, all wrapped up with an inclusive and gender-neutral bow. In two years, Tanaya has built a thriving community that provides a safe place where no topic is too taboo to talk about!

In whatever free time she has left, Tanaya likes to hang out with her rescue dog Samosa, pretends she can read Latin, and scuba dives and eats her way around the world.

T0054609

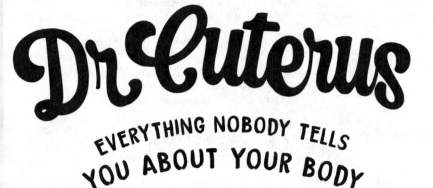

Dr Cuterus

EVERYTHING NOBODY TELLS YOU ABOUT YOUR BODY

✳

DR TANAYA NARENDRA

PENGUIN BOOKS

An imprint of Penguin Random House

PENGUIN BOOKS

USA | Canada | UK | Ireland | Australia
New Zealand | India | South Africa | China

Penguin Books is part of the Penguin Random House group of companies
whose addresses can be found at global.penguinrandomhouse.com

Published by Penguin Random House India Pvt. Ltd
4th Floor, Capital Tower 1, MG Road,
Gurugram 122 002, Haryana, India

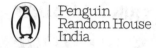

First published in Penguin Books by Penguin Random House India 2022

Copyright © Dr Tanaya Narendra 2022

All rights reserved

10 9 8 7 6 5 4 3

The views and opinions expressed in this book are the author's own and the facts
are as reported by him which have been verified to the extent possible, and the
publishers are not in any way liable for the same.

ISBN 9780143455707

Typeset in Adobe Caslon Pro by Manipal Technologies Limited, Manipal

This book is sold subject to the condition that it shall not, by way of trade
or otherwise, be lent, resold, hired out, or otherwise circulated without the
publisher's prior consent in any form of binding or cover other than that in
which it is published and without a similar condition including this condition
being imposed on the subsequent purchaser.

www.penguin.co.in

Contents

FOETUS DELETUS

OHEMGEE! WHAT'S WRONG WITH ME?!

Wel'cum'!

About This Book

This is not a book about sex.

I mean, it won't teach you how to have sex. It's not like . . . an instruction manual.

Instead, this is a book that introduces you to your body. Especially those parts that we don't frequently talk about. Y'know, the stuff hidden inside your pants. And then, what you decide to do with those parts—whether you smash them up against someone else's parts, or you keep them nicely hidden away inside your pants . . . well, that's entirely up to you. But we reaaaally need to talk about those parts. We need to talk about your genitals, your so-called 'private parts', because without them, we wouldn't be here. I'm not joking, after all, you were born only after your parents smashed their own genitals together (ick, I know, but it is a fact of life!).

You can think of this book like that extrovert friend who introduces you to all their other friends, and then you have friends of your own. It's your party book that makes you cooler than all your friends. (Okay seriously, just mug up some cool facts from here and try them at your next party. You're gonna be such a hit!) This book will reach inside your pants, bring out your genitals (I mean, not literally) and introduce you to them, in the hopes that you become good friends. Because even though we collectively decided at some point that our body parts will be 'haww' and not 'aww', I would like to help you change that. Cuz your genitals are really aww (I'm not called Cuterus for nothing).

Other than ensuring the continued existence of humanity, our genitals do a lot for us. Like, a fuck ton (no pun intended). They're involved in peeing, perioding, and pleasure (solo, or with a partner). The last point is especially important because —Trivia Time! —human beings are among some of the only animals in the world that have sex for pleasure. Dolphins (who, contrary to popular opinion, are actually not that cute, and like to rape other animals for fun) and bonobos (who are actually pretty cute but super horny) are the only other animals who have sex for pleasure. Anyway, all these functions I just mentioned are pretty important. So, why don't we talk about them? Why are genitals hidden in the dark corners (I mean, it's important to keep them wrapped up for legal reasons) when they're actually so cool? We'll delve into some of that and also talk about the stuff on the inside. We will talk about your internal organs, how they are linked with your outside stuff, and the cool things they do, and the things that can go wrong. Let's put on our nerd glasses and get super sciency, because we'll be discussing your 'genitourinary system'!

But wait, there is more.

We will also talk about all things sex—safety, precautions, pregnancy, how to get pregnant, how not to get pregnant, infections, consent—phew, that's a lot.

There is still more.

Basically, there is a whole lot you're going to learn about your body, science, history, politics, and marketing. This is the kind of book you should display on the coffee table at home to show off to people that you're so cool. And yes, I am appreciating my own book, but as you'll find out, it is bloody awesome (JUST LIKE YOUR BODY!).

So, let's start off, shall we? Like every good play, we will first begin by introducing the characters. So, friends, it's time to meet your body!

Meet Your Genitals

Hello there! It's time to meet your body!

I'm hoping you're already a little familiar with your body. You have inhabited it for at least a few years and probably already know well that weird backache that starts for no reason, that stray chin hair that sprouts no matter how frequently you pluck it out, and that one stupid pimple that keeps saying hello even after you pop it.

But do you know about your sexy bits? The parts that we don't discuss so publicly? The parts you want to learn about but are afraid of Googling or asking someone? I mean, sure, you've awkwardly discussed your genitals with your friends with a lot of giggling. And maybe you've seen some porn and been confused about how your body parts look in comparison to the porn stars. Maybe you've even managed to study the infamous reproduction chapter in your biology textbook, and learnt about some of the very technical aspects of reproduction . . . but do you really *know* about your body?

Now, obviously, you know your body way better than anyone else can ever tell you. But our sex education and body education are so technical that, frankly speaking, it's a bit boring. Okay let's be real, it's very boring. Nobody remembers (or even cares about) the epididymis, or the fimbriae on the

Fallopian tube. But instead of looking at all this from a boring, technical angle, let's see it from a more flattering angle: you see, sex is fantastic, our sexy-time bits are fantastic, and we have oddly been hiding these fantastic things in shame for ages. So, put on your nerd hats, roll up our sleeves, and get this sex ed party started!

Woohoo!

Okay, so:

1. How many ovaries do women have?
   A) One
   B) Two
   C) Eight
2. The female equivalent of a penis is:
   A) The vagina
   B) The ovary
   C) The clitoris
3. The average length of an erect penis is:
   A) 14 inches
   B) 5.1 inches
   C) 2 inches
4. Mitochondria is:
   A) The powerhouse of the cell
   B) The powerhouse of the Dell
   C) The most useless piece of information you know

Okay, so the answers are:

1B, 2C, 3B, 4C. How did you score?

I believe in you, and I know you've aced that quiz! So, give yourself a well-deserved pat on the back, and let's move ahead because things are about to get really interesting. You are about to meet your genitals.

Before we move forward, one basic thing to establish is how sex and gender are different things. We'll learn more about this later, but for now, let's understand that your genitals don't define your gender. Gender is about your identity, and how you feel; whereas sex is about your chromosomes and the genitalia you were born with.

Coming back to your body parts and that much-awaited genital introduction: You can understand these organs in two broad ways—the sexual organs and the reproductive organs. The sexual organs, i.e., the clitoris, vulva, vagina, penis, help during the sexy times whereas the reproductive organs, which are the uterus, ovaries, testicles, penis, help in the baby-making times. Some people also like to classify them as internal organs or the ones you don't see versus the external organs or the parts you do see. The classification doesn't make a difference because I am not going to make you take an exam on this (just short quizzes, lol) but it's just nice to divide it into two broad areas, so you have some context.

Because beauty starts on the inside or some crap like that, I thought it might be great to start with our internal organs. The ones that stay hidden away under folds of your skin, and are usually involved in the baby-making task. Y'know, the stuff you should have learned about in school in the reproduction chapter but your teacher awkwardly skipped through it. And we'll start with the star of the show . . . the uterus (dude, my name is Cuterus for a reason; I sincerely love the uterus).

It's Your Bits

1

The Uterus

The plural of uterus is uteri, which sounds like a someone with a Bhojpuri accent saying, 'You try', and which is super sassy because try as much as you can, you can NEVER be as cool as the uterus. Seriously, just look at it.

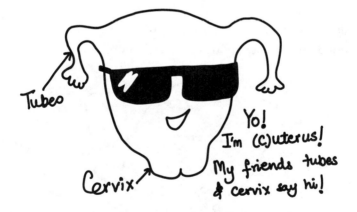

Uterus wearing sunglasses and looking cool

Textbooks, very boringly, describe it as a 'hollow, pear shaped, fibromuscular organ', which basically means that . . . it's a hollow organ (d-uh), that is shaped like an upside-down pear, and it's made of a lot of muscles (*dolay-sholay*) and fibrous tissue. In fact, it's one of the most muscular organs in the whole body! A great way to think of it is that it's like a balloon. It's shaped like a deflated balloon. It can expand like a balloon. And it can hold a lot inside it, just like a balloon. And the uterus is super fun, just like balloons! (Although it turns out, balloons are terrible for the environment. My childhood died when I learnt that sad fact.)

Now the uterus has one job that it takes very very seriously and is shockingly good at it. The job is to accept the baby, nurture it and then violently push it out when the baby is old enough—a little bit like what your parents did. The uterus is our OG parent, *Jagat Mata*. For the most part of its life, the uterus lives inside your pelvis. Except when it's pregnant and filled with the baby + baby juice, when it grows massive and extends all the way up into your abdomen.

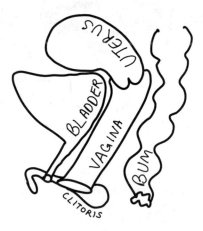

How other organs fit around the uterus

The upper part of it hangs on top of your bladder, kinda like it's piggybacking on it. That's why pregnant people need to pee so much—the massive uterus crushes the bladder under its enormous weight, and the bladder can barely hold on to any pee. Right behind the uterus, you've got your colon. No, not the perfume that your man applies, that's cologne. I'm talking about your colon, the intestine. The shit that holds your shit. More specifically, right behind your uterus is your rectum.

Tanaya's Trivia Timeout!

Because of how the uterus lives near the rectum, some people experience this really sharp, funny pain in the butt when they are on their periods. Us science nerds call this pain Proctalgia Fugax—proct = butt, algia = pain, fugax = shy or fleeting. So, it's shy butt pain! Don't ask me why it's called that. Medicine is weird!

So that's the Google Maps location of your uterus. *Bladder ke peeche waali gali mein, rectum se ek ghar aage.* But what exactly does it do? Can you be born without it? What does it have to do with your periods? And pregnancy? SO MANY QUESTIONS!

Okay, easy there, tiger. Let's get into all of this, one by one. The first being what does the uterus do. Well, it's really very simple. The uterus is your first home, ever. That's where you start life, as a teeny tiny cluster of cells, tightly gripping onto the walls of the uterus. This is where you find nourishment, grow, and become a teeny tiny creature with a head the size of a football. The uterus protects you inside your mum, absorbing all the shocks, jerks, and movement. You know, like an airbag in a car. When you are old enough and the time is right, it creates a series of contractions to eventually push you out, and safely deliver you into the hands of a doctor, who will give you a tight slap on your bum bum. Doctors aren't sadists—this is just to get you to scream, so your airways can clear and you can breathe like a normal human being. Instead of leeching oxygen and nutrition off your mum, like a parasite. So, basically, the uterus has the function of accepting, and nurturing a pregnancy, when it happens.

And when this pregnancy doesn't happen, the uterus has the function of screaming BLOODY MURDER. This is not an analogy; I legitimately mean blood and cramps and pain. Now, the reason why this happens is that your uterus really wants to get pregnant. All the time. So much so, that it builds a lining on the inside, kinda like skin but on the inside. This layer is called the endometrium: endo meaning inside, metra meaning uterus. (It's also the joke I text my mom to let her know when I am able to find space in the metro.) It's all about the pregnancy for the uterus. So anyway, it keeps building up the endometrium on the inside, to make it nice and soft and cosy for the baby when it comes in. Now obviously, you are not getting pregnant every single month (can you IMAGINE what the world's population would be like if that were to happen), which means your uterus gets uhhh . . . angry. It gets angry and then it throws out everything it has built up inside. The nice and thick and fleshy endometrium goes straight out of your uterus, through the cervix, into the vagina, and out of your body. And that's a period! Doctors jokingly call it 'the weeping of a disappointed uterus', but if you have a uterus you'd know that it's not a joke, because periods can really be painful.

There are two reasons why periods are painful, and both have to do with this habit of your uterus of squeezing itself like a lemon to let all the blood out. Our body creates these fascinating chemicals called 'prostaglandins' that work on juicing your uterus to get the period blood out. Because there is only a small hole through which the blood and mucus as well as all the extra tissue inside in your endometrium can exit, the uterus requires some extra help. The prostaglandins help by squeezing your uterus to effectively get more blood and tissue out. Because of this squeezy situation, the blood supply to the uterus gets cut off every few seconds. This causes more pain. And that makes your period feel like hell.

Now uteri sound like an endless nightmare of pain and blood, so is it possible that you simply can't or don't have one? Well, yes, as it turns out. In a rather rare congenital disorder called Mayer Rokitansky Kuster Hauser (MRKH) syndrome, people can be born without a uterus or with an underdeveloped uterus. That sentence must have been very difficult to read out aloud. Let me explain. So, a congenital disorder is something that you are born with. It usually occurs when something goes wrong during development, when you are still growing inside the uterus, which we call in-utero. MRKH is a rare condition in which the uterus, the vagina, and/or parts of them may be underdeveloped or completely absent. This obviously creates a problem with the whole period and pregnancy thing, which is how it's often diagnosed. When young girls haven't had a period until the age of 16, this is one of the things we look for. This is because people with MRKH usually have 'normal' looking external genitalia, so most people don't suspect they might be born with whole organs missing. There are lots of treatment options depending on how much is underdeveloped and missing, and so it's different for different people. Most people with MRKH also have functional ovaries, which means they may be able to have their own biological children through techniques like in vitro fertilization (IVF). And that leads me to a brilliant segue: say hello to your ovaries!

2

The Ovaries

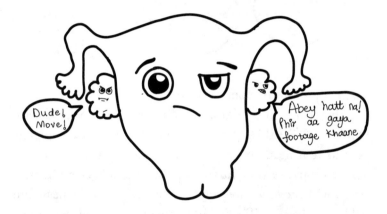

Okay. We might have to zoom in. Let's check the uterus out from behind to see better. We'll go towards the back of the uterus and try to spot the ovaries from there.

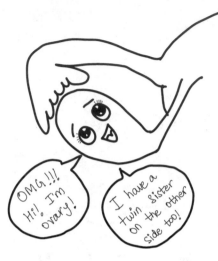

Aaaaaand, those are your ovaries!

They hang out next to, but slightly behind, your uterus. Think of it like this—let's say your ears are not completely fixed to your head and can move around a little. If someone attached ropes to your ears and pulled them back a bit, your ears would move a tiny way to the back of your head but still be on the side. That's kinda how your ovaries are placed near your uterus. Contrary to popular opinion, they are not actually attached to the Fallopian tubes. The tubes just hover over your ovaries, like a party hat. You've got one ovary on either side and they are the VIPs of your pelvis, because they have some really important functions.

These important little organs are quite small—they're about the size and shape of an almond! I had to go hold an almond in the middle of typing this sentence because it always amazes me that something so small controls so much about the existence of our species on this planet! From these almond-sized miracles, we get oocytes. An oocyte, aside from being a very fun word to say over and over— ooooocyte!—is basically an egg, which when it fuses with a sperm, makes a little baby. The ovaries are the real *murgis* of your body (okay, let's be polite and not call them chickens). They are female gonads, aka glands with a reproductive function; men's gonads are the testicles. They not only make the eggs and keep them safe until you can use them, but also produce some very important hormones, estrogen and progesterone. These hormones regulate a lot of things in our bodies, like developing boobs, periods, how good your skin is, pregnancy, and overall health.

A really cool thing about your ovaries is that they contain all the eggs you are ever going to have. Unlike men, who produce new sperm regularly, women do not infinitely keep producing new eggs throughout their lives. You are born with a limited supply of eggs in a lifetime, and this is why it gets harder to get pregnant as you grow older. Basically, think of it like this: you are moving into a new house, and that house has 40,000 eggs. You enjoy making omelettes for breakfast, and your survival relies on you eating omelettes for breakfast. (Omelettes are really important in this analogy.) But because this house only has 40,000 eggs, you can only make 40,000 omelettes. Or maybe only 38,789 omelettes as some eggs will turn out rotten, some will break, and some will make omelettes that you put too much salt in and then you have to throw out. After some 38,789 days, no matter how much you love your omelettes, you unfortunately will not be able to make any more of them. It is the same for making babies.

You see, we have a limited supply of eggs that we are born with. Every month, our body selects a couple of dozen eggs and provides them with nutrition, so they become big and strong. Out of these dozen eggs, one grows to be the biggest and strongest, which is then released in the hopes of making a baby. So, we spend a lot of our egg-related allowance each month for this baby-making madness. The body tries to push out the best-quality eggs early on, and keeps the poorer quality ones in the back, hoping we don't have to use them for our omelette, err . . . baby-making process. Naturally, and sadly, as we grow older, we have fewer and fewer eggs, and lower in quality too, remaining, which means that, unfortunately, delaying your pregnancy *too* much is not the best idea. You want to make your omelettes, and you wanna make them fast.

Actually, if you're not ready to make your omelettes yet, you could just freeze them. Egg freezing is a technique that allows you to freeze your eggs and plan a pregnancy later. This can be done for medical reasons—such as cancer treatment, since most cancer chemotherapy drugs can damage the eggs inside your ovaries—or for social reasons, such as if you're not in the position to plan a pregnancy right now. Egg freezing enjoys a modest success rate of 30–40 per cent at most places, and is quite an expensive process. If you are an employee at Apple or Facebook, they might help you cover the cost for it! Trans men can also choose to freeze their eggs in case they want to have a biological child from their own eggs in the future, using IVF and surrogacy.

All in all, nature really did us dirty with that whole biological clock bullshit. In order to hurry us up on the reproduction front, human beings developed so as to be obsessed with baby mania, and to try to have them at some point in their lives. We are, unfortunately, evolutionarily geared towards really loving making babies. The survival of our species through many millennia has rested on our ability to make many cute, screaming little ones. This, especially, is ridiculously interesting when you think about the fact that because women are born with all the eggs they will ever have, you would also have been a tiny egg inside your grandma when she was pregnant with your mom! This Russian doll situation is probably a bit complicated to understand like that, so let me explain:

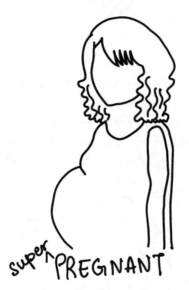

super PREGNANT

Let's imagine this is your grandma when she was pregnant with your mom. Let's zoom into her tummy, her uterus to be more precise.

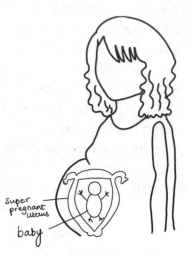

super
pregnant
uterus

baby

See, that's your mom when she was a teeny tiny baby, inside your grandma's uterus. Now, remember how a baby girl is born with all the eggs she will ever have in her life? This means that your mom, in this baby form inside your grandma's uterus, contained all the eggs she would ever have in her ovaries.

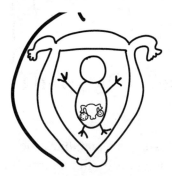

Look at your mom inside your grandma's uterus. And look at all the little eggs in your mom's tiny foetus ovaries, those dots inside the baby ovary are eggs. One of those tiny dots is you. After your mom was born, she grew up and had those eggs mature, and one of them was fertilized by your dad's sperm, and then became YOU. The egg that created you was already formed inside your mom when she was a baby inside your grandmom. So, your grandma quite literally carried you too. Isn't that wild? Two generations inside one human!

When a girl is born, she has around 2 million eggs in her ovaries. And while that may sound like a lot of eggs, it's actually really not because for some bizarre reason, most of the eggs die before you're ready to use them. By the time you hit puberty, aka when you are old enough to make babies— we all know 12-year-olds are not old enough to make babies but that's basically what puberty is—you will only have about 400,000 of these eggs left. Just 4–5 lakh out of the 20 lakh. What is this cruelty, Nature *Mataji*? First you send us in with an already limited supply of eggs, and then you take commission from that tiny amount too?

Unfair eggspectations aside, we need to talk about how your body gets ready to even make these omelettes. Let's talk about puberty. Or more specifically, how your ovaries help you get to puberty. You must definitely have heard of estrogen and progesterone. But what do they actually do? And why do we have to talk about them right now? Well, this is where the other function of your ovaries comes into play— they make hormones. They make estrogen, progesterone, testosterone (wait, isn't that the 'male' hormone? Yes, but women need it too!), other androgens, and some more fancy stuff we don't need to remember because I am totally not taking a quiz on this later (muhahaha). These hormones help you in growing and in going through puberty. Estrogen is the sexy hormone: It helps you develop boobs and a juicy butt, among other things. This is also the hormone that is more active during the first half of your menstrual cycle (but more on that later), which is probably why you feel great and your skin looks fantastic right after you finish your period. Progesterone is the preggo hormone: It helps your body support and nourish a pregnancy. This is what comes in during the second half of your menstrual cycle (and yes, more on that later) and helps maintain a nice, thicc, juicy endometrium for a baby to implant in. Together, these hormones along with several others help you navigate the incredibly stormy term in your life called puberty. They help you grow, sexually mature, and maintain your sexy and baby-making bits all through your life.

All this doing their job stuff is well and good, but sometimes, like every unruly teenager, your ovaries misbehave and produce cysts. These cysts are of two main kinds: functional cysts, the ones that are formed as a side effect of normal everyday functioning of the ovaries, or non-functional ones, which are the bad guys, from polycystic ovary syndrome (PCOS), endometriosis, or even ovarian cancer. Most ovarian cysts are not cancerous; however, the risk of a cyst being cancerous goes up if you are older. Non-functional cysts can make your ovaries really huge, and sometimes they can twist over on themselves in a dangerous condition called ovarian torsion. Think of it like your ovary acting like a cute ballerina and pirouetting inside your pelvis, leading to a not-so-cute emergency situation. This is usually marked with incredible pain, vomitting, and feeling pretty shit. You'll need emergency surgery if you have a torsion. The opposite happens as you grow older and hit menopause, when your ovaries shrivel up in size instead. Your omelette-making capacities reduce, and the ovaries stop releasing eggs. It is then that menopause hits, and it begins a new revolution of hormonal clusterfucks in your life.

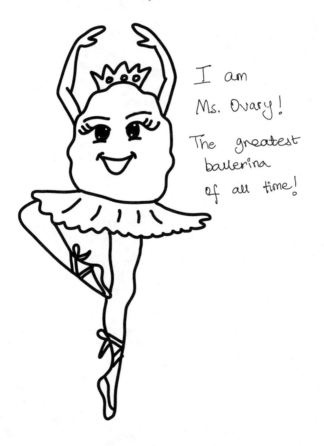

Basically, your ovaries do a lot for you, and they're very sweet and cuddly little balls that deserve more love than we give them. Your brovaries really love you. It's time we love them back.

3

The Vulva

Will the real vulva please stand up? I repeat, will the real vulva please stand up? We're gonna have a problem here.

Imagine teaching your children that the nose is actually called the mouth, and never telling them what a nose is. How will they know anything about the nose? How will they ask the right questions? How will they tell the doctor they have a problem in their nose? And how will they know how to describe their problem if there is a problem in their nose if they think that their nose is called their mouth? Sounds confusing? And stupid? It is.

We have all had a massive identity crisis when it comes to our genitals—most of us, almost all of us, in fact, have called the vulva the vagina our whole lives. 'I'm going to shave my vagina' (dear God, the horror of stuffing razor blades INSIDE your body); 'I have vaginal darkness (HOW? How can you have darkness INSIDE your body?); 'Vaginal wash' (have you ever put soap inside your nose? Why would you put it INSIDE your genitals?)—my relentless use of the capitalized 'INSIDE' should probably remind you of the fact that the vagina is the canal inside the body. It's the long tunnel inside the hole between our legs. It's not the stuff on the outside. It's not where pubic hair grows. It's not the part that is in contact with our clothing, it's not what you see when you see someone's downstairs area . . . all of that is, in fact, your vulva.

I have plenty of thoughts about this so I wrote a whole paragraph on it. But first, I need to explain what a vulva is; you can find my angry rant at the end of this chapter.

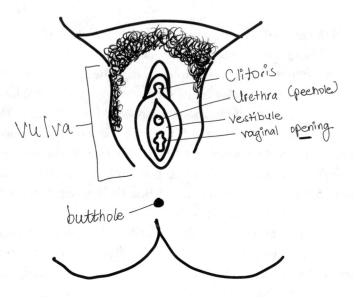

For now, it's time to meet your fantastic, glorious, beautiful vulva—this is your external sexy-time parts. Vulva in Latin means 'covering', which is a great way to remember that the vulva is the outside covering, and the vag(i)na is the thing on the inside. Starting from the top, you have the mons pubis (the pubic mountain), some people also call this the FUPA or fat upper pussy area, which is the fatty part on the top; labia, these are the fleshy 'lips' that you see when you look at someone's genitals; the clitoris, the little pea-sized pleasure centre; and when you part the lips, you have the urethra (the pee hole), and the vaginal opening. It also contains some glands that help you during sexy times. Between all of these and the butthole, you have a small area called the perineum.

The mons pubis or the FUPA is actually present over both pussies and penises, but it's fatter above the pussy—that's because it acts as a cushion to protect your pubic bone when you're doing the sexy times. Once you hit puberty, this part gets covered in a luscious bush of pubic hair (which we will talk about in another chapter). If you go down (pun intended) from the mons pubis, you come to the labia. These are the lips—outer (labia majora) and inner (labia minora). The outer labia are smooth and have hair on them. The inner labia usually look shrivelled up like a raisin and can hang outside, or be completely covered by, your outer labia. Your mons pubis, and especially your labia, can be darker than the rest of your body. This is because when you hit puberty, your skin starts producing more melanin, a pigment that gives your skin its colour and protects you from sun damage, in these areas and your underarms. And that's how your skin gets darker around your genitals and in the underarm area, not because you shaved!

The vulva is also, strangely, the focus of a lot of beauty rituals, a whole multi-trillion-dollar industry worth of things. Washing your vulva; grooming your pubic hair; dyeing your pubic hair, or even getting pubic hair wigs; vajazzling or decorating your vulva with plastic stick-on crystals; yoni

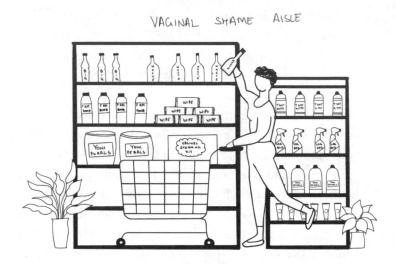

pearls; lightening your vulva; using perfumes for your 'vaginal area'; getting vulva facials, hilariously called vajacials or vagina facials; vagina tattooing or vattooing, which just sounds silly; surgery to change the appearance of your labia; and vaginal steaming are just some of the rather questionable treatments available for your vagina (they mean the vulva, but you already know that).

But the real question is, are any of these things even required? What happens in these procedures? Are they safe? Let's take them on, one by one, and you'll soon realize how much pressure there is on our vulva, comfortably hidden inside our pants, to match up to some very unrealistic beauty standards. Vulvas are naturally more pigmented, wrinkly, hairy, and have a natural smell. There is nothing wrong with any of these things. Yet, we have managed to build a complicated beauty routine to 'fix' these issues.

I'm going to start with the most annoying and widely used category—vaginal washes. First off, you do NOT need to wash your vagina. Leave it alone! The vagina cleans up after itself (unlike your disgusting ex). As my personal hero, star gynaecologist and author Dr Jen Gunter, says, 'Cleaning inside the vagina is like cigarettes for your vagina.' Second, while you can use a gentle wash to clean your *vulva*, plain water is fine too. A lot of these products do tend to make some very tall claims—pH balancing, being dermatologist tested, and what not. Ignore all that. You cannot balance the pH of your vagina by applying something on your vulva. Also, take a look at the ingredients—tea tree oil, fragrance, dyes, essential oils, and alcohol are common additives in 'vaginal' washes, which can be irritants for a lot of people. Such products can cause dryness, irritation, allergies, and if inserted internally, can also cause pH changes, disrupt the natural bacterial colony in your vagina, and, therefore, put you at an increased risk of sexually transmitted infections (STIs).

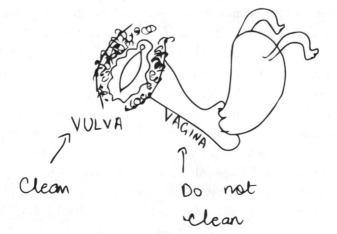

VULVA

VAGINA

Clean

Do not clean

If you do want to use regular soap externally, a simple glycerine soap, mild vulva washes, or even something like Cetaphil, or a fragrance-free gentle face wash for eczema-prone skin are great options. Or skip the whole ordeal and just use your hands and water. Make sure to *gently* clean the folds, especially between the labia majora and minora, and around the clitoral hood. You might find some white gunk that you can easily remove with your finger—don't worry, that is just debris and dirt that is a result of, well, existing. Don't be harsh. Don't use heavily perfumed soaps or soaps containing glitter. Don't put anything inside the vagina. That's it, that's literally all you need. There is no need to build this mega trillion-dollar industry into something bigger, but if you like using a wash and it's worked for you so far, then go for it!

Something to notice is how the messaging behind many of the feminine hygiene products is just . . . dirty. You've heard me say this a thousand times, but your vagina and vulva are meant to be the way they are. They do not need to smell like a spa. And they are NOT dirty or smelly contrary to what advertising might tell you. And using these products will not make you 'pure' and 'fresh' (you and your crotch are not a loaf of bread that will go stale). There is also the larger issue to consider that if your vagina/vulva/discharge actually does smell bad, then it could be a sign of infection and you would require medical care. Just masking it with some perfume will not suffice. You should be going to the doctor. Also, why are we unnecessarily gendering this? Trans and non-binary people also need to maintain hygiene, right? And why is this marketing so selective and targeted? Have you ever seen a penis deodorant on the shelves? I don't like putting my money in the hands of companies that use such shady marketing tactics to sell their products—it's shameful, disgusting, and unethical.

Two products that personally exasperate me to no end are wipes and perfumes for down there. Not only are these vulva wipes entirely unnecessary, they are bad for the environment and, depending on the ingredients, they are probably bad for your vulva too. I had a patient who would clean herself so aggressively with wipes after going to the gym that she developed rashes and constant irritation on her delicate genital skin, and needed long-term medication to help her recover. Sometimes, such chronic irritation can cause scarring and permanent damage. Many of these wipes contain alcohol, which dries out your delicate skin; tea tree oil, an irritant; and added fragrance, which are not just unnecessary but actively harmful for a lot of people. You don't need to clean yourself with a wipe all the time; a simple shower will do the job and you really don't need those intimate wipes (unless, of course, you can't have a shower and clean up).

With all that said, if you do like using it and it has posed no problems, you can continue using it as long as you do it gently. My approach to fragrances for down there is not so relaxed—you should strictly not be using it because, repeat after me, your crotch is not smelly or dirty. And if it is actually smelly, you should see a doctor, and not irritate your skin with fragrance and postpone seeking medical care for treatable issues that can be easily resolved instead of waiting for them to get complicated.

Okay, let's pause for Trivia Time, because you need to know the story behind why I get so angry about this and you should too. You see, women, vulvas, and vaginas have been blamed for all of humanity's ills since the beginning of time—Eve ate the apple, Pandora opened the box, periods and labour pains are the price we pay for our womanly sins, and the vagina is so inherently dirty that most of our cuss words revolve around being a pussy, or being fucked like a pussy. The marketing and ideology behind products for hygiene down there often tie into this larger narrative. It's good ol' historical misogyny masquerading as feminine hygiene products.

Did you know that Lizol (your *pocha-waala* Lizol) was originally marketed (as Lysol in the US) to women to get rid of 'odours' and help preserve 'marital bliss'? These guys legitimately insinuated that the smell of vaginas was ENDING marriages across the world, and that using Lizol inside of your vagina would help CURE the smell?! Yeah, this is the same bathroom disinfectant that we use now, except it was much worse, because back in the day, the formula was stronger—it could cause pains, burns, poisoning, and even death. Not just Lizol, but Listerine (the mouthwash) was marketed for the same purpose. Washing the inside of the vagina is a practice known as douching, which has been linked to having twice as high a likelihood of causing ovarian cancer versus not douching, this is aside from many other health risks of douching such as increased risk of STIs and pregnancy complications. Ditch the douche, dude.

Then there is the highly convoluted process of manicuring your pubic hair, which, you should know, does not need to be removed—we have a variety of contraptions

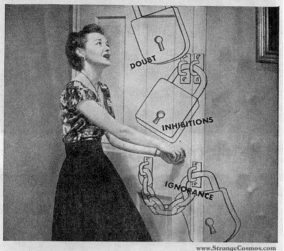

to manage it and give it errr . . . hairstyles. It goes further: into pubic hair colouring, modelling it into specific shapes, and adding crystals all around, called vajazzling. If you are not satisfied with your own pubic hair, you can also buy pubic hair wigs online that come in a variety of colours, textures, and shapes. They are called 'merkins' and were used historically by women who would remove their pubic hair to protect themselves from pubic lice (yes, you can get lice aka *jooein* in your pubes) and by sex workers to hide any evidence of genital diseases from STIs. These days, merkins have an interesting role in films—when actors have to do nude or semi-nude scenes, they just use merkins like a robe to cover their genitals from unwanted exposure—how cute! There is a huge variety of merkins available, which are made from synthetic or real human hair, and they come in a variety of textures and colours!

Tanaya's Trivia Timeout!

Before we had antibiotics, some STIs, like syphilis, were treated with mercury! Mercury, as we know, is kinda poisonous, and has an interesting side effect of causing baldness—not just on your head but also in your pubic region. And thus, merkins became the absolute height of syphilis chic. Love is in the hair, after all.

Okay, now that we've removed all the hair, the underlying skin is exposed—the normally pigmented underlying skin, especially in us Indians. And not surprisingly, considering our obsession with skin whitening, we have built a huge industry around whitening our genitals. But here is the doctor's advice—there is no reason to use any creams or lotions, or get any expensive treatments, to lighten this natural pigmentation. This pigmentation occurs at puberty and is literally a sign of sexual maturity—so why would you want to remove this sign of maturity and have your genitals resemble a baby's? That's obviously not sexy, is it? Not only is it completely unnecessary, but these lotions and creams often contain exfoliating acids that can damage the fragile skin of your genitals, cause significant pain, and get this . . . lead to more pigmentation! One of the ways in which our skin heals itself is by increasing pigmentation in the damaged area—that's why scars are always darker than the surrounding skin—which makes this whole affair counter-intuitive. You don't need to lighten your skin anywhere—not your face, not your genitals. That stuff is bullshit and dangerous.

Some of the more light-hearted practices embraced by this industry are getting vaginal (VULVAL) facials, and temporary tattoos (ouch), which I guess is okay and fun? I mean, pamper your kitty, I guess? As long as they are not using strong exfoliation on your genital skin, a little facial could even be fun. You might think that the same could be said about vaginal steaming (and once again we scream 'vulva!'), which can be a fun little spa experience, except it can actually be quite harmful. The idea is based on the premise that you go to a fancy (read expensive), spa to squat over a pot of boiling water containing some herbs that claims to 'cleanse' and 'detoxify' your vagina and uterus, and cure a whole host of issues, including depression and infertility. BUT (*a*) your vagina is self-cleaning, (*b*) detoxing, unless medically mandated for things like addiction, is bullshit, because your liver, lungs, and kidneys do it for you anyway, and (*c*) there is this rather important question of how exactly the steam is going to go all the way into your uterus and vagina when you are only steaming your vulva. Like, can you steam someone's door and say you've steamed their whole house? It just doesn't make any sense! On top of all this, did you know that you are more likely and more quick to get burnt by steam as opposed to hot water? By adding constant heat and moisture, you are also creating ripe conditions for the growth of fungal infections. To this, add the risk of having an allergic reaction to the herbs in the mix, and you have a perfect cocktail called Don't-Steam-Your-Vagina-Mar(*khaao*)garita. Your vagina is not a wrinkled suit that needs steam ironing. While there are several health benefits that certain herbs and foods can have on your overall health, using them to steam your vulva is not the way to get those benefits. Am I saying that vaginal steaming has no actual benefit other than very temporarily increasing blood flow to your vulva (which you can also do by just putting a hot pack between your legs) but can also be harmful? Very harmful? Why, yes! You are a quick learner.

Some people also like to opt for surgery to change the appearance of their vulva. Now while this is great if you have medical reasons, such as your labia being so long that you accidentally sit on them and hurt yourself, I'm really not a fan of 'cosmetic' surgery for purely 'cosmetic' reasons simply because our ideas of what is cosmetically appealing have changed so much and so often throughout history that it's not just a waste of money, but it's also upholding weird beauty standards that are pretty useless. All in all, your hairy, bumpy, wrinkly, dark vulva is meant to be like that. And you don't need to change it.

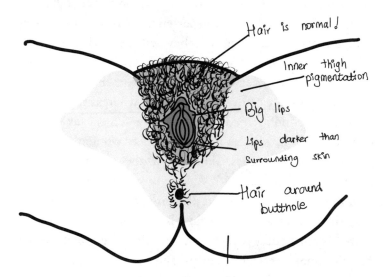

Now, it might seem pedantic—we all know what we mean when we say, 'I'm gonna shave my vagina'—but we know that nobody is putting a razor inside themselves. But allow me to go on a little feminist rant here: it's important we call it the right name, not just for biology class points, but because it has bigger implications. You wouldn't like it if you were named Shreya, but everyone called by you your sister's name, Shruti. Not only is that annoying, it's also incorrect. The term 'vagina' has been used to refer to all of the female genitalia since forever and it actually reduces the already tiny amount of attention that female health issues generally get. It's as simple as how you cannot educate people or raise money for testicular cancer if you keep calling it penile cancer. Also, it's no surprise that women have fewer orgasms compared to men when we don't even tell them where exactly it is that we experience pleasure—if we keep telling them it's the vagina, they will keep thinking that penetration alone is going to make them orgasm! It's this constant erasure of sexual pleasure for women—the vulva is where the pleasure centres are (clitoris!) whereas the vagina is involved in childbirth and reproductive-centric sex (penises go into vaginas), which somehow reduces women to just . . . vessels to make babies. That's not the motivating force behind our existence, is it? We are more than baby-making factories, and our health and pleasure DESERVE focus and attention. Especially in a world where men consistently have more orgasms and get more pleasure from sex than women do, it's important we put our pleasure on the map.

To conclude: What are the top five tips for a happy vulva?

- Wear breathable cotton underwear, and don't sit in sweaty clothes or swimsuits for too long
- Wash with water (and/or a mild, gentle soap)
- Don't douche, use wipes down there, or vulva deodorants
- Rock the pubes! If you must remove them, then trim instead of completely getting rid of them
- Sleep without underwear (no seriously!)

VIVA LA VULVA!

Note: People who have had gender-affirming surgery and have surgically created vaginas are medically required to douche, as their neo vaginas don't have the same self-cleansing mechanisms.

4

The Vagina

The vagina has a very strange and interesting history. We have ignored it so completely throughout history that we didn't even have the word vagina until Gabrielle Folloppio, the same guy after whom the Fallopian tubes are named, decided to call it 'vagina'. And this was actually an improvement on the old term—originally, all of the female external genitalia were referred to as pudendum. This will hurt really badly when you hear what it means: Pudendum comes from the Latin word 'pudenda', which means something to be ashamed of. Yeah, the name of our genitals literally meant something to be ashamed of. The father of Greek medicine, Galen, thought the female sexual organs were a 'deformed' penis. The dude legit thought the vagina was an inside out penis, like a sock.

The vagina is not something to be ashamed of. I want to change that. The vagina is genius! The vagenius, if you will. Language matters a lot, and I want to rename my vagina something that reflects how cool it is. So, I want to introduce you to a reimagined vagina—the supercool, marvellous organ that sits inside your pelvis. Meet Vajayanti. She is an A-list celebrity that the paparazzi loves to stalk but actually has zero idea about. Vajayanti is your typical old-time heroine—greatly misunderstood but packing a real juicy story on the inside! Just like many of the biggest stars who are very private about their inner lives, so is Vajayanti. She prefers to stay indoors, stylishly *pardanasheen*, wearing the cover of the hymen like a pair of dark sunglasses to keep herself even more private.

She lives in the apartment right below her friend, Urethra, in the very posh and exclusive locality between the two labia. You can see the main door of her house from the outside, always shielded by fancy curtains imported from Hymenland. When you step inside, you see she is a party girl who parties hard with her friends—Mr Penis, Ms Tampons, Mx Sex Toys, and Ms Menstrual Cups. She's very graceful, always wearing a sari (we'll understand this in a second), which makes sense as she's quite tall, long, and muscular. You see, Vajayanti, or your vagina, is the tunnel that connects your uterus to the outside world. The vagina is simply a canal, not the whole external genitalia. We sometimes refer to all of the lady bits as the 'vaginal area' but that's as accurate as calling your cheek the 'ear area'.

The long vaginal canal has a door on either side; the vaginal opening on the outside and the cervix on the inside. If you think of your uterus as a palace, then the vagina is the long driveway, the cervix is the main gate of the palace, and the labia are the gates of the driveway. This controls whatever goes in or out of the vagina.

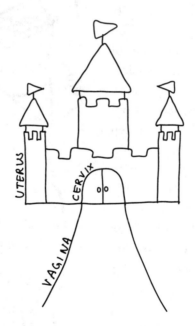

Actually, it's not quite a canal, as in it's not always expanded and it is not open at all times. Most of the time, the walls of the vagina are touching each other, like a deflated balloon. When you are aroused, this deflated balloon opens up, increases in depth, and secretes a slippery substance that makes you wet. Well, a lubricating substance is always secreted by Vajayanti, whether or not you are aroused. It's a combination of fluids coming from the cervix, the lubricating glands around your vagina, some dead cells, and some fluid leaking from the vaginal walls. This is known as vaginal discharge and it helps keep your vagina healthy and clean.

Think of it like Vajayanti's skin care—vaginal discharge is like expensive serum, the vaginal version of that fancy hyaluronic acid you use to keep your skin plump. You start producing vaginal discharge at puberty, and continue secreting it all through your life until menopause. After menopause, the vaginal discharge often dries up, which can lead to a lot of issues like vaginal dryness, recurrent UTIs, and experiencing pain during sexual intercourse. This discharge is super important! Normal vaginal discharge can be clear to white in colour, has a mild odour but shouldn't smell bad, and changes in consistency through the month, sometimes being thin and at other times being thick and sticky. If at any point your discharge suddenly changes colour—becomes yellow, green, red or grey—or has a strong odour, or is accompanied by itching, burning, or pain, you should see your doctor. This could be an infection. But regular, everyday vaginal discharge does not need to be 'treated' and it is essential for good vaginal health.

As we have learnt, douching is BAD, and washing Vajayanti from inside can change her pH. Normally, the vagina has an acidic pH (similar to beer and wine). This is important because the vagina is full of good bacteria on the inside, which work as your internal defence army, protecting you from bad microorganisms. Vajayanti is full of a bacteria called lactobacilli, the same good bacteria found in yogurt, that produce lactic acid and keep the vagina acidic. Most infection-causing microorganisms don't like an acidic environment, so having a tangy environment prevents their growth and keeps your vagina healthy. This is how your vagina keeps itself clean—it is self-cleaning and takes care of itself! Soap is basic, the opposite of acidic, so using soap inside the vagina can alter the pH. The natural acidity also causes those bleached parts on your panties—you know, those weird orange or light-coloured patches that develop in your underwear. Vaginal discharge is so powerful that it bleaches the fabric of your underwear! In fact, this same acidity is responsible for causing brown blood towards the start and end of your period. Because we release such a small amount of blood at these times, the vagina oxidizes or digests the iron in the blood, making it turn brown, just like when iron gets rusty. I told you, Vajayanti is badass.

Now, Vajayanti is a classy lady—she is powerful, graceful, keeps herself well groomed and clean at all times . . . but she has terrible posture. Vajayanti doesn't stand straight with an erect spine, instead she always leans back. The vagina is not a straight canal, but is actually directed backwards. If you were to draw an arrow starting from the vaginal opening all the way to the top of the vagina, it would not be pointing straight upwards, but instead be tilted and pointing backwards towards your butt. This is why it can feel like you're hitting a wall when inserting a menstrual cup or tampon. Just tilt it back, pointing towards your butt, and it should go in much more easily.

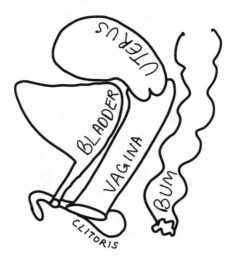

Terrible posture aside, Vajayanti's pretty chilled out. She hangs out on a hammock of muscles all day, looking and feeling fabulous. This hammock of muscles is called your pelvic floor. Imagine your pelvis to be like a big picnic basket holding your organs, which are like fruits inside it. In order to make sure the fruits stay inside the basket, you need a strong basket floor. Your pelvic floor acts the same way; it keeps your fruits (organs) like the uterus, vagina, bladder, and rectum safely inside it. Pelvic floor muscle weakness can lead to a number of health issues, such as urine leakage and pain during peeing or sexual intercourse. So, in order to support Vajayanti and her friends, we need a strong pelvic floor.

The word 'vagina' actually comes from Latin, and it literally means a sheath. This is really, well, dumb, because it implies that the vagina is a sheath for the penis sword. It makes it sound like a vagina is just a passive ditch that exists to please a penis. Actually, our Vajayanti is more like an enthusiastic athlete who is actively involved in sexy times. When you are 'turned on', you literally turn on a rush of blood to your pelvis. Your clitoris swells with blood and becomes erect (just like a penis!); your vulva starts looking darker; Vajayanti begins 'sweating', that is, the vagina starts releasing a clear fluid through its walls to add lubrication. Small glands at the entrance of the vagina, called Bartholin Glands, also release a fluid to help with lubrication. As this isn't a pregnancy book, I won't get into a lot of details about vaginas during pregnancy and labour. But here's a fact: When giving birth, the vagina can expand up to 300 per cent in size to shoot out a giant baby, and then promptly return to its original size in six to twelve weeks. Vaginas are not passive.

So, unlike what Galen thought, Vajayanti is not some deformed penis, but is actually really cool. Now, Vajayanti has to deal with a whole lot of body shaming, as people seem to have a lot to say about the size of the vagina. Is it too big? Is it baggy? Is it loose? Well, it is big, yes. It's important for our vaginas to be big, and to be able to expand even further. Before someone with a penis gives themselves too much credit for their ginormous organ and the resulting necessity of a vagina to be expandable, let me stop you in your tracks. Ever thought that vaginas NEED to be big, because we need to, you know, push a whole human out of there? Humans have exceptionally large brains—the very brains that have enabled us to come up with preposterous ideas such as 'the vagina becomes loose from sex'—which makes it necessary to have a large birth passage. And so, human vaginas developed to become more like an expandable suitcase that can become larger to accommodate more things inside it. When you are sexually aroused, the vagina opens up and becomes deeper, to make space for a penis to go inside it. In the same way, it needs to become larger and wider for a coconut-sized baby head to go through it.

You can think of your vagina like a sari. A sari is actually 6 metres long, but you can fold it up into a 1 foot by 1 foot square that fits neatly inside your cupboard. The vagina is similar as it has loads of tissue inside, which is usually neatly folded up and available to spread out whenever required. If you stick your fingers inside your vagina, you will be able to feel many ridges and folds. This is just to help increase the surface area, the same way your brain also has a lot of ridges and folds to increase the surface area. Vajayanti is a highly elastic organ, with a huge surface area that has evolved to fit into a small space inside your pelvis. Your stomach also works the same way, with several folds inside it to make it expandable. If you eat too much food in one sitting, no one ever says your stomach will become loose. Then, how can we say that having sex can make your vagina loose? It's simply factually incorrect.

Also, I love how people suggest that having sex with the same penis over and over and over again is perfectly okay for keeping Vajayanti tight but having sex with different penises makes her loose. How the hell does that work? Vajayanti isn't moulding around the penis, literally changing herself to perfectly match the penis every time you have sex. And by this logic, wouldn't sex then make the penis shrink? Maybe these are the real questions to ask. (Just kidding, shaming any one for the genitals is not okay.)

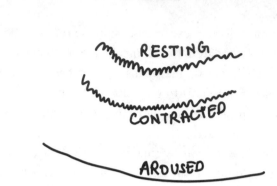

While sex doesn't change Vajayanti's size, it can definitely make her gassy. This is especially likely to happen if you are having sex doggie style, or if you're exercising. You might have experienced a 'prrrrbt' sound coming out of your vagina sometime—Vajayanti has musical aspirations, y'all. This 'farting' sound coming from your vagina is called a queef. But it's actually not a fart; it's just trapped air rushing out of the vagina and making a noise. It's the vaginal equivalent of making a fart sound with your mouth; it is like the sound of air rushing out of a balloon. On the other hand, a fart happens when food is digested in our intestines by our gut microorganisms and some smelly gasses are produced as a result. A queef is not a fart, but just an air pocket. It's nothing to be embarrassed about and instead is something you can heartily laugh about with your partner. Or maybe you can share a sweet chuckle just with Vajayanti. She's your friend, after all.

Okay, farting aside, does Vajayanti pee? So, we don't actually pee from our vaginas. There is a separate hole in vagina owners, called a urethra, from where we pee. This tiny hole is visible right above the vaginal opening. This is why you are able to pee comfortably while wearing a menstrual cup or a tampon; the vagina is where these products go in, and the peeing happens from the urethra. I told you, Vajayanti's a classy lady.

Call it whatever you like: pussy, cunt, vagina, pudendum, penis fly trap, vajayjay, Vajayanti, or whatever name you want to honour it with—the vagina is badass. It punches out all the bad guys and keeps itself healthy, it has superhero-level strength and pushes out whole babies. It regularly carries out it's skin care routine, is super intelligent, and is damn lovely. Your vagina really is a star.

5

The Hymen

Many people believe you lose yours when you say 'hi men!'

Sorry, that was the lamest joke in this book, but you know those are the only ones I'm good at. Although, on a serious note, many people really do believe you somehow actually 'lose' a whole piece of tissue from your body when you have sex for the first time. What a *kamaal*! The disappearing magical unicorn! You may have an inkling now that this is a myth we're going to bust, and you probably have many thoughts popping up in your head—so many questions, so many myths, so many assumptions about this teeny, tiny piece of tissue in our bodies. So, let's write an entire chapter on it, obviously.

What is the hymen though? Like, is it this seal that locks our vaginas, keeping us sacred and pure until we have sex for the first time? Is it a holy marker of our virginity? Is it the most important *dhakkan* in our bodies? Well, you probably know that I'm going to say that that's a load of unscientific bullshit, because that *is* a load of unscientific bullshit. Because what the hymen actually is, is just a thin membrane that exists around the vaginal opening, partly covering it. It even means 'membrane' in Greek, that's how membranous it is. It's located at the entrance of the vagina, about a centimetre deep, and looks pale pink or white in colour. Some people like to be fancy and call it the vaginal corona instead of the hymen—'corona' means crown—but I really don't think any of us have positive associations with that word post 2020, so we will continue calling it hi-men. Oops, I mean, hymen.

Where the hell is the hymen anyway? Let's take a look at the vulva.

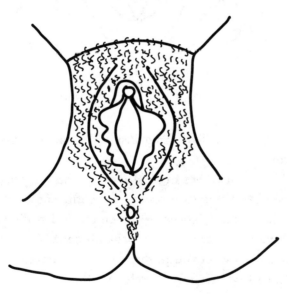

Okay maybe let's zoom in a bit. I'll remove the pubic hair so you can see better.

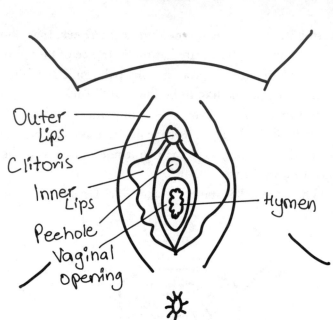

That rubber band-like thing inside the vaginal opening is the hymen.

Waise toh, it comes in all shapes and sizes, it most often is shaped like a ring surrounding the entire entrance; or like a half moon, partly covering the entrance. I really want to sing '*Mere vagina waali khidki mein ek chaand ka tukda rehta hai*' but I don't want you to throw away my amazing book in disgust, so I will restrain myself. Another type of hymen is where the membrane has two holes, with a thick band, called a septum, going through the middle. Think of it like your nose. Your nose has two nostrils, which are basically just holes with this thick thing between them. Incidentally, this thick nose thing is also called a septum. I will spare you the surprise and tell you that in medical terms, a septum means a wall; so now if you see septum or septate anywhere, you can put on your nerdy glasses and do some *doctoribaazi*. Sometimes, this hymen can actually be covering the entire entrance to the vagina, much like a *dhakkan*, but that's a complication we will talk about later.

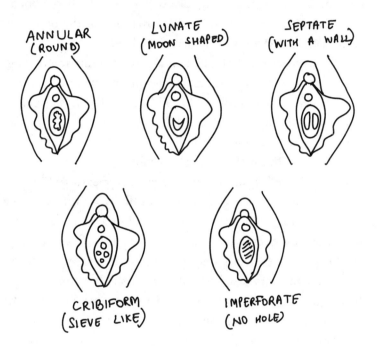

Actually, no . . . wait, it's too interesting to leave for later. Some hymens *completely* cover the entrance to the vagina, like a door. One of the things that can happen in such hymens is that they have many little holes in them. They're more like a *chhanni*, or a sieve, as opposed to a *dhakkan*. After all, you are a human being, not a tetrapak. Or, more interestingly and bizarrely, sometimes these hymens may have absolutely no tiny perforations in them either, very well making you a tetra pak. In this situation, since the vagina is completely blocked, menstrual blood cannot leave the body. It's in such conditions that doctors need to come perform some *khul ja sim sim* surgery and actively make a cut into the hymen so the period blood can leave the body. So, all I'm saying is, a completely sealed hymen is not the best idea. And that's not what most hymens look like.

The development of a hymen is actually quite interesting. When you are a teeny, tiny tot inside your mother's uterus, the vagina develops like a solid tube. Think of it like a sausage: it's long and cylinder shaped, and filled with stuff on the inside. Eventually, during intrauterine life, i.e., when you are still a teeny, tiny tot inside the uterus, this solid tube starts to become hollow—the cells from the inside start disappearing. Think of it like the cardboard insert in a toilet roll—your future vagina starts evolving into something resembling that cardboard insert, so it's hollow on the inside. Starting from the top, all the inside cells start disappearing and then move down. However, the very last layer of cells at the bottom manages to stay behind, looking almost like a sheet, and becomes the hymen. So, it's just like that little piece of toilet paper that you forgot to remove from your toilet roll, except it's covering one of the ends of the toilet roll and is not on the body. That's how we get a hymen.

Other than humans, whales, elephants, chimpanzees, and horses have hymens, but it has no importance in their lives. Which brings me to my next question: If the hymen doesn't actually mean anything, then err . . . What does it do? Why is it there? To be honest, I'm not sure how to answer that question, because I'm not sure I know the answer. We have no idea why the hymen exists. There is no known biological function of the hymen! Scientists and doctors just go 'huh' when asked why this develops in the first place. Some research suggests that it's meant to protect the delicate vagina when we are younger, since in our early years, the vagina is basically just an open tube with none of the sophisticated self-protection machinery that comes in later as we grow older. So, it's probably meant to be like a shield when we are babies, and just meant to act as a physical barrier in place of the vaginal army of good bacteria that comes in when we're older. But again, we have nooooo idea if that's what it really does. That's just what we think it does. Sounds plausible, though? I guess. We think it pretty much does nothing.

So now that we know what it does, which is probably nothing, it's time we talk about why it's so hyped up. Why do we hold the hymen in such high value? Does the tearing of the hymen actually mean anything? To answer that question, I'm going to start by blowing your mind (yes, once again) with a really cool fact: The hymen actually has very few blood vessels. Which means that when injured, it really won't bleed a lot. So, often, 'bleeding' from a 'torn' hymen might actually be blood from lacerations and internal injuries inside the vagina. Technically, even when it does 'tear', there should only be a little bleed. In fact, studies show us that 40–60 per cent women reportedly do not bleed when having sex for the first time— which is half of all women! Some cultures have a horrifying practice where the sheets are examined the morning after the 'first night' to check for bloodstains and ensure that the bride was a virgin. When, most often, these bloodstains would be the result of terrified young girls bleeding vaginally from lack of natural lubrication. See, here is the magical thing—your vagina is really pretty cool. When you are sexually aroused, your vagina automatically expands to allow the entry of a penis (and the hymen, at the entrance of the vagina, also stretches and relaxes with it to allow this entry). On top of this, it also releases some natural lubrication, to smoothen the entry of the penis and avoid pain. This just makes the vagina slippery, the same way that putting soap on your hands before you take off the bangles that may be too tight for you adds slickness. If you force something into an unlubricated, unaroused vagina (and unrelaxed hymen), it's only natural that it will cause injuries that bleed. This has been confused with '*seal todna*' and 'popping the cherry' for many sad years.

In fact, there is so much stigma around this issue that some people resort to getting surgery called hymenoplasty or hymenorrhaphy before having sex or before their wedding night, to make sure they bleed when they do have sex. In this (rather stupidly named) 'revirginization' surgery, doctors reconstruct this membranous tissue so people can become 'virgins again' by having a hymen. Obviously, a lot of people find this hugely problematic as, if you remember, the hymen actually has no medical value. Having or not having a hymen does not make you a virgin. (Or unvirgin? Devirgin? What's the correct term?). Unfortunately, apart from surgery, there are more 'fake hymens' available for purchase online, which can be inserted vaginally and 'bleed' when penetrated. But once again, I will remind you that not everyone bleeds when they have penetrative sex for the first time, and you can hurt and injure your hymen in many other ways too. Inserting things like tampons or fingers, horse riding, or even vigorous stretching can cause your hymen to tear. As a matter of fact, most penetrative sex can leave your hymen intact. According to a few studies, some women examined during CHILDBIRTH were found to have whole-ass hymens in their vaginas. And they obviously did not become pregnant magically by some strange divine intervention.

Sadly, virginity tests and hymen checks are still carried out by doctors and medical institutions. The idea is to check if someone has ever had sexual intercourse by examining their hymen. This is hilariously dumb because during our entire medical education, doctors don't receive any training on how to look at a hymen and conclude whether or not this person is a 'virgin'. How are doctors going around diagnosing something that not only means nothing, but about which we have no training to diagnose anything? Doesn't sound very scientific to me. Not just that, having your bodily autonomy violated in this way is horrifying and demeaning. The controversial 'two-finger test' involves inserting two fingers into someone's vagina to see if they can accommodate those fingers comfortably. Not only is this super objective and reductive, but it's also inaccurate—you simply cannot determine someone's 'virginity' by looking at their vagina and hymen. Additionally, as mentioned, the hymen can rupture in many other ways besides sex and some people can even be born without a hymen! The two-finger test is an unethical, unscientific, humiliating, and harmful practice. The act of someone inserting their fingers into any body cavity (as anyone who has ever had a colonoscopy or their butt examined by a doctor will tell you) can feel oddly intimate. To have that done on the grounds of proving your 'pureness', when that very idea is built on such flimsy and inaccurate evidence, is truly wrongful. Thankfully, many countries have banned the practice now. In 2018, the World Health Organization (WHO) published a report roundly condemning this practice. The honourable Supreme Court of India even called the test 'hypothetical', pointing out how this test can be invasive and undignified for the person going through it, which really makes me want to dance sometimes because it's so great that our highest legal institution recognizes how illogical this test is.

TL;DR: Hymens ≠ virginity.
(Virginity is a social construct anyway!)

6

The Clitoris

Okay, the chapter on this tiny pea-sized little thing might be the biggest and most interesting chapter in this whole book, because it's *so* much more than the *matar ka daana* you think it is.

Wait, let's rewind for a second. What the hell am I even talking about? There is a high possibility you might not even know what this organ is. Okay then, prepare your mind to be blown because you're about to meet the coolest organ in your body—the only organ that has no other reason for existing other than for giving you pleasure. Yepp, you read that right.

This organ was born for one job, and damn, it really understood the assignment, because it takes your pleasure very seriously, even if you don't. Meet the Clitoris.

Iske ghar ka naam Clit hai, waise you can call it whatever you want.

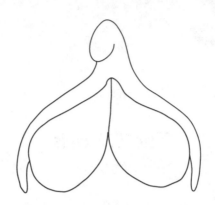

Ummm . . . okay so that probably doesn't look like anything you've seen before. Also, I know I said the clit is a small pea-sized thing. This doesn't look pea sized or even pea shaped. Errrr, excuse you, but what the hell. Okay, let's see if this looks more familiar. Probably more like it?

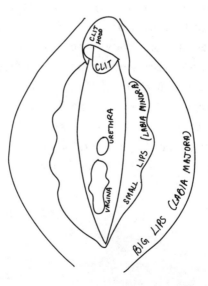

Yeah, we don't actually see the whole clitoris when we look between our legs. That's why we think of it more like a *matar ka daana*. It's actually more of an iceberg situation, where you only see a tiny part but the *Titanic*-killer is actually much bigger underwater.

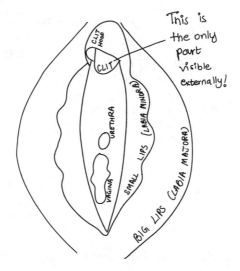

And while that's the only part visible externally, the whole clitoris, as you now know, is much bigger. A lot of it is internal and it extends all the way behind your labia. Let's do a full clitoris course: first, we will understand the geography and topography, then move on to the history, and then go down to the business administration end of things. We'll begin with some magic! Let's remove the colour from the top part of this diagram, so you can get a behind-the-scenes, special backstage pass and see what's happening in the VIP lounge:

You see how the clitoris lies behind most of what you see on the vulva? That's why pressure in this general area can feel so good (okay I'm getting ahead of myself, we'll learn this in the MBA Clitoris section). Anyway, here is the whole clitoris, in all its glory:

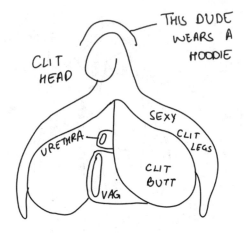

It straddles the vagina and urethra (pee hole) between its thick fleshy parts, called the body of the clitoris, which actually looks like a cute butt. It's also got these extensions, which I call sexy clitoris legs, that extend down from its head. Okay, let's call them clitoris arms, maybe, because otherwise it's hella weird to imagine. The head is covered by a hood (just like you wear a little hoodie in the winter) because it is super, super, super sensitive. Trivia Time! You'll see lots of internet articles saying that the clitoris head contains 8,000 nerve endings, but that's not exactly true. This number was based on analysing a cow's clitoris. (Yes, cows have clitorises too. Also, hyenas have megaclitorises that they give birth from . . . okay getting ahead of myself again. I know a lot of animal clitoris facts and they're really cool and I can't wait to share them with you . . . AND OKAY, TANAYA GET BACK TO THE TOPIC.) We're not entirely sure if humans have the same number of nerve endings on their clitorises. Some people also say the clitoris has twice the number of nerve endings compared with a penis, but again, we don't know if that's true. It's possible that they are more densely packed on a clitoris, but we're not sure if they're double in number. We'll probably need to examine some human clitorises before we can come up with a definitive number, but as you will learn through the chapter, history and science have not been kind to the clitoris. The question of why the hell though continues to baffle me because clitorises are seriously cool organs.

Now that we have a basic understanding of where the clitoris lies and what it looks like, let's delve into some history. Not the boring, battle kind, but the interesting history of how the clitoris develops in your body to become the kickass kickasser it is. Let's do some baby talk, then. No, not the *ale mela babu khaana khaya* type. The embryology type, aka the study of embryos or the teeny, tiny babies inside a uterus. Let's start with the most mind-blowing bit: When we are wee little things inside our Mum's uteri, for the first few weeks, all of our bodies develop the same way—as females! (Yes, the original blueprint for human development happens to be female.) Now, depending on what kind of building instructions you come with, i.e., your chromosomes or your DNA, you can either be XX (female) or XY (male), or intersex (different variations of X and Y combinations). If you are XX, it's pretty chill and you continue developing the same way. But if you're an XY, some time in the ninth week, your body suddenly wakes up and it's like, 'Bro, I need to make some testosterone', and suddenly goes into testosterone overdrive. And this is where the fun stuff happens. Testosterone comes over with a magic wand and transforms that original 'female' blueprint you were following. What was developing as the ovary becomes the testicle (wuttt!), parts of the vulva (the big lips) become the ball sack (aka the sack in which testicles live), and get this, what was developing as the clitoris, BECOMES THE PENIS! Whaaaaaatttt! The 'female' equivalent of the penis is not the vagina! But the clitoris! Isn't this so crazy and so cool? I actually like to call the penis an overgrown clitoris, but I am a radical clitoris fan. What's even stranger and cooler is that when you are turned on the clitoris becomes erect the same way a penis does. Such organs are called homologous. So, the clitoris and the penis are homologues. We will learn about a lot of homologous organs in other chapters, but for now, that concludes (for the first time ever in human history) our fun section on the history of anything!

So, now that we know all the intense biology, let's talk about its executive functions: what exactly does the clitoris do? And why am I so hyped up about it? Is it something very special? Why is it so special? And wait, if we're talking about pleasure, how are we missing the conversation about the G-spot? Okay, deep breath, because your mind is about to be blown! As I mentioned earlier, the clitoris is packed with nerve endings and is the only organ in the human body that exists *solely* for the purpose of sexual pleasure. Rubbing, tapping, or stimulating it directly using fingers, the mouth, toys, or the penis, and even indirectly stimulating it with penetration, are great ways to enjoy sexual pleasure via the clitoris. Which can usually lead to an orgasm! (And orgasms are GREAT for your health. Not only do they feel fantastic but also do all kinds of good things for your heart health, for your skin, for your stress levels, and just overall wellness).

But how do these awesome orgasms work? And are vaginal orgasms better in some way compared to the ones from the clitoris? Whatever you've read about 'vaginal' orgasms being more 'mature' versus 'clitoral' orgasms being more 'immature' is 100 per cent bullshit, because all orgasms come from the clitoris (most probably, we're like 99.99 per cent sure). This mature versus immature orgasm theory was just a myth perpetrated by an Austrian psychoanalyst called Dr Freud. He had a lot of really weird theories, such as the Oedipus complex and the Electra complex. (Please Google this because it's really very intriguing and I need to get back to the clitoris.) And, get this, most people (like more than 75 per cent people who have a vagina—report having orgasms from stimulating the clitoris and not from penetration. The realllllly fun part (I know I keep hyping this up so much but it's legitimately that cool) is that the G-spot may probably not even exist and is probably just the clitoris! (Again, most probably. We're 99.99 per cent sure.)

Okay this obviously begs the question, what *is* the G-spot? You might have seen or heard about this famous unicorn magic button located somewhere inside your vagina that supposedly miraculously makes you orgasm every time you touch it, and you've probably spent a significant amount of time wondering where it is inside you, and whether you are broken because maybe you don't have one? Named after a German dude gynaecologist called Dr Gräfenberg, the supposed location of the G-spot is 2–3 inches deep, on the anterior vaginal wall, aka the front (or top wall) of your vagina. Some researchers even think that this is a female prostate. When I was younger, I was obsessed with romance novels that described how the hero would make the heroine experience the absolute pinnacles of ecstasy by giving love to her magical G-spot. Obviously, I then indulged in some serious *Pirates of the Caribbean*-style treasure hunting looking for my G-spot, only to end up feeling dejected about the absence of my magic orgasm button. Internet articles, magazines, books, movies, even sex toys, all seem to be obsessed with the G-spot. But the truth of the matter is that *maybe* the G-spot doesn't even exist.

If you do stick your fingers inside yourself or your partner and curl your fingers up, you end up stimulating the top part of the vaginal wall, and you might notice that this feels more pleasurable than touching other parts of the vagina. This is the supposed location of the G-spot, and it's really hard to stimulate this particular area with a penis, although fingers and sex toys do the job well! But does this mean that touching this area will automatically lead to intense toe-curling orgasms? Most likely, no. And since we mentioned that the clitoris is responsible for orgasms, does this mean that this is separate from the clitoris? Also, most likely, no. See, the thing is, most researchers and sexologists think that the alleged G-spot is actually just your internal clitoris. Remember how we saw that the body of the clitoris sits on the vaginal canal like you would sit on a horse? It's very likely that the G-spot is just the area between the legs of the clitoris that indirectly gets stimulated on stimulating the top wall of the vagina. It's kinda like if you covered your legs in a thick blanket and then proceeded to rub your clit from over it, would it feel good? Sure! Will it lead to an orgasm? Probably not. So, it's obviously completely normal that most people orgasm purely from pleasuring the clitoris.

This area of research is so complex and ever evolving that science has come up with a new name called the 'clitourethrovaginal complex' or CUV complex and before you freak out about the length of the word we'll break it down to understand it better: the clitoris + urethra + vagina together make up something really cool, and this area where all three of these organs intersect seems to be the home for pleasure. So instead of running after some legendary button like the G-spot, let's just understand that the clitoris, urethra, and vagina work together via the CUV complex to help us orgasm, whether from penetration or not. This area has even been visualized using imaging techniques such as magnetic resonance imaging (MRI)! So, this means that the clitoris has a huge role to play in orgasms, the urethra is also somehow involved, and the vagina is more than just a passive . . . sock that exists just to accommodate the penis. I like this theory. It makes sense to me.

There are also some theories that hold that if the vagina were so highly innervated, i.e., having so many nerve endings, then childbirth would become impossibly painful, and women would just say NO to sex and pregnancy. So, making the vagina orgasm-central may not be the best approach for making sex appealing. And making sex appealing has been a really big priority during evolution so that we make lots of little babies and ensure the survival of humanity (*baap re*, so much pressure on our little shoulders).

As you've seen throughout this chapter, the clitoris has been largely ignored, hidden, run away from, had myths and the like built around it throughout history . . . I mean, it wasn't even until 2009 that someone actually made a 3D rendition of what the clitoris is shaped like. That's how badly we treat women's sexual health and pleasure. So, it's okay if you have a vagina and you don't orgasm from penetrative sex. Most vagina people don't. It's okay if you need to give your clitoris a genie-inducing-style rub to have an orgasm. This is totally normal. You're totally normal.

And you don't need to fake that orgasm for your partner.

Last piece of *gyaan*: Show your partner how you like to be touched instead of faking it. This will make you both happy! And happy, healthy people are all we want!

7

Boobs

Have you ever wondered how blue whales feed their babies underwater? Of course, you haven't, you only think about yourself. 1. That's a joke, and 2. Of course, you do; who else will otherwise! But seriously, how do blue whales feed baby blue whales underwater? Won't all the milk get mixed with sea water? Now you may never have thought of it, but whale boobs are a marvel of nature: a single boob is 1.5 m or 4.9 ft long, and weighs as much as a baby elephant. Whale boobs are the largest boobs on Earth. They produce 200 litres of milk every day, containing almost 50 per cent fat. It's the consistency of toothpaste, which is how baby whales can slurp the thicc milk easily, even underwater. But these boobies are hidden inside the blue whale's body, in folds of skin called 'mammary slits'. It's like an in-built flesh bra. When they're hungry, babies go under the mommy whale and nudge at the slits, and the mommy whales stick their nipples out, squirting milk straight into the baby whale's mouth. I told you, blue whale boobs are a marvel of nature.

In contrast, human boobs are very, well, different. We've got these beautiful little globs of fat and glands sitting proudly on our chests, all day every day since puberty. Unlike other animals, human boobs have the distinct pleasure of being permanent; once you develop them, they never quite go away. Scientists are not quite sure why this happens, but we have several theories: our boobs become boobilicious at puberty to indicate that we are now sexually mature; our boobs developed to help our babies grab onto something while we hold them at our hips; our boobs developed as fat stores to tide us over in times of starvation and so on. Whatever theory you want to believe in, our hooters are really damn interesting. They look great, they're super cute and squishy, and they make milk which sustains us in our early years. Boobs are hella important and cool. I mean, we are called mammals because we have mammary glands. But like all the other bits in our body, no one really ever teaches us about our boobies. So, what are boobs anyway?

Boobs, the technical term being 'breasts', are teardrop-shaped fatty glands that all mammals have on their chest. For all the other 5,000 mammals besides humans, boobs become larger at the time of ovulation—the animal equivalent of sexy red lipstick to let them know you'd be down to getting naughty—or when they are nursing their newborns (boobs = milk factory). Humans develop them at the time of puberty, and they not only make milk for nursing their newborns, but also have a social and sexual role. Now breasts have three main parts: the 'breasty' part of the breast, the areola part, and the nipple. You can understand this better if you think of a cupcake. Imagine the cake part of the cupcake is the actual breast. The icing on top is the areola, the dark skin surrounding your nipple, and the cherry on top of the cupcake is the nipple. They're also like cupcakes in the way that they are delicious, cute, and come in a variety of shapes, sizes, and colours. Internally, breasts are made up of fat, structural tissue, and the milk-making gland parts. The percentage of all these internal parts is variable and dictates the size of your breast.

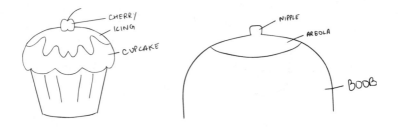

And that relates to the biggest concern about our breasts . . . their size. We tend to fret a lot about the size and shape of our breasts: too small, too big, not perky enough, too perky, too droopy. If your breasts are even slightly large, they will sag. This is a fact of life because this is how gravity works. If you stick two large bags of sand to a wall, they will hang down like boobs do; and just like the bags of sand, your breasts cannot defy gravity. Some people like to wear a push-up bra to temporarily defy gravity, the keyword being 'temporarily'. With that said, wearing a bra does not prevent sagging, and not wearing a bra does not make your boobs saggy. Oh, and on that note, wearing underwired bras, bras at night while you sleep, or black bras will not give you breast cancer. Using underarm deodorant too will not give you breast cancer. Bras are more of a fashion statement than anything else, but some people with heavier breasts find that wearing bras makes them more comfortable and prevents under-boob sweat (or as they say poetically, humidititties). Big or small, wearing or not wearing a bra is 100 per cent your choice. If you're a trans woman, wearing a bra can feel gender-affirming. If you are a trans man, binding your chest instead of wearing a bra can be very gender-affirming. Our boobies mean different things to different people. And the boobs themselves have great diversity!

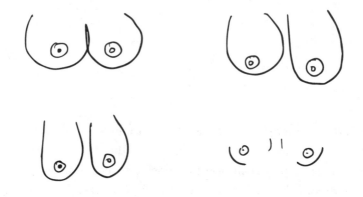

Our built-in milk jugs come in all shapes and sizes; in fact, two breasts on the same person can be of different sizes. Most people reportedly have a larger left boob (did you peek into your shirt when you read this? No shame, I did too) compared to their right, and this inter-boob difference can be as big as one cup size. If you read the testicle chapter (Chapter 8), you'll know that testicles also have this same issue. Our bodies are not very symmetrical, so it's totally normal to experience this with any paired body part. Aside from this, breast size also fluctuates constantly throughout your life, depending on how your hormones have decided to behave on a particular day. You can expect a more dramatic change in size at puberty, when breasts begin to develop; during pregnancy, when your body is getting ready to activate its milk production capability; during lactation (d-uh); and during menopause, when your breasts might shrink a bit as they don't need to be making milkshakes any longer. Some people also find that their breasts become larger and tender right before their periods, when they are PMSing. We think this occurs because in anticipation of a pregnancy, our hormones 'turn on' the milk production factory in the boobs which makes them suddenly grow larger. Additionally, our bodies hold on to more water before our periods—which is why you might also find your weight goes up when you're PMSing—but this is yet to be proven scientifically. Either way, your boobs might feel sore and look more boobilicious when you're PMSing. Your breasts will also change size if you gain or lose weight since a large part of our breast is made up of fat.

Interestingly, your breasts blow up when you're aroused, just like the testicles, by up to 25 per cent. Aside from an increase in size, your nipples also become erect, the veins on the boob skin become more prominent, and you might see a darkening of your areola. In fact, the breasts, areola, and nipples—which fancy scientists call the breast–nipple–area complex—can be highly sensual and very sensitive to touch. Some people can even experience nipple orgasms, or nipplegasms. This works because your brain has an area called the genital sensory cortex, which is 'turned on' (teehee) by stimulating the clitoris, vagina, and, you guessed it, the nipples. If you haven't experienced it, don't worry, there isn't anything wrong with you, not everyone can experience nipple orgasms. But nipple play can be pleasurable for most

people, of all genders; so go ahead and lick, flick, and kiss
your partner's nipple as they are likely to really enjoy it!

While most of us only have a pair of nipples, some
lucky people have more than two nipples! The extra ones
are called supernumerary nipples, and can range from one
extra nipple all the way to eight extras! Either way, they
are nothing to be worried about as they just are something
left over from our development when we are embryos.
Irrespective of how many you might have, your nipples can
also come in a variety of shapes. Some people have nipples
that point outwards, some have flat nipples, and some have
nipples that are almost buried inside the areola. These are
called retracted nipples. As long as your nipples have always
been like that, this is totally okay; our bodies come in a huge
variety. However, if you notice any sudden change in the
shape or colour of your nipples and areola, then it's a good
idea to see your doctor. A sudden change in the way your
nipple looks could be a clue to underlying diseases, and the
earlier it is diagnosed, the better.

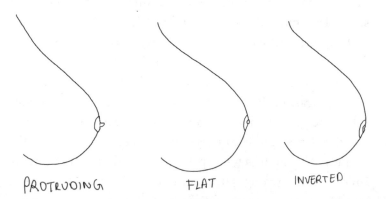

PROTRUDING   FLAT   INVERTED

We mistakenly call the whole darker part the nipple, when actually only that little nub that sticks out is the nipple. The rest of it is the areola. While you may only have seen light-coloured areolas in porn or on TV, areola can come in a wide variety of colours. In us Indians, it tends to be darker: ranging all the way from a pale wheatish brown to a deep brown to even almost black. You may also notice your nipples becoming darker after pregnancy and delivery because of a change in hormones. Humans have a beautiful diversity in our nipples and areola; you absolutely do not need a fairness cream to lighten their colour. I promise. Companies that sell such products thrive on making you insecure about regular features of your body and then attempt to sell you a 'cure' by preying on your insecurity. That cure doesn't work and can sometimes contain very harsh ingredients that damage skin and can lead to long-term side effects.

Aside from being a beautiful chocolatey colour, your nipples and areola can also have hair growing around them. We humans are hairy creatures, so this is normal; feel free to tweeze these out if it bothers you. I've just learnt to embrace my furry body, nipple hair and all, as otherwise I'd constantly be walking around with a pair of tweezers. You also might see some raised dots along the edge of your areola: They are called Tubercles of Montgomery and they secrete a sebum, or natural moisturizer, to keep your boob skin moisturized. If you have ever breastfed, you'll know that this sebum is super important. Having a very cute little parasite attached to your tit, constantly draining you of all your milk and energy, can often irritate the nipple and lead to nipple soreness. Babies can sometimes accidentally or (on purpose) bite your nipples, so that's some added joy. Moisturizing and soothing nipple creams can offer some relief from this horror.

But how do breasts work anyway? Like how does this whole breastfeeding system work? Let's take a look inside the boob to understand this. If you were to slice open a boob like a cake, you'll see an interesting arrangement inside that looks like this:

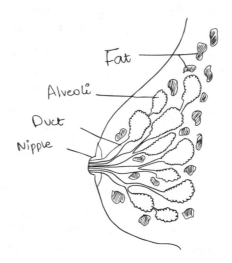

The fillers are bits of fat, which influence the size of your breasts, and all those pathways that you see leading up to the nipples are called ducts. These ducts connect the nipple to the alveoli, which are the grape-like clusters you see on the inside. Fun Fact: You also have similar looking alveoli inside your lungs, where the gas exchange takes place—oxygen is added to your blood, letting out the carbon dioxide! The word 'alveoli' basically means a small cavity. So, the two chest bags you have, whether 'inside' meaning your lungs, or 'outside'

meaning your breasts, are quite similar! They both contain little bags. Milk is manufactured inside the breast alveoli, and the ducts take it towards your nipple. When a baby suckles on these nipples, signals go into your brain which instruct your nipples to release the milk, and that's how you breastfeed.

This organic, biodegradable packaging *waala* human milk is pretty cool: it contains antibodies, vitamins, minerals, carbohydrates, fats, and proteins—all of the good stuff. In fact, this breast milk is pretty intelligent too as its composition changes with the age of the baby. In the beginning, it is antibody-rich to help develop the baby's immunity, and later, the milk becomes more nutrient-rich to ensure good growth for the baby. It also contains a lot of good bacteria for good baby gut health and good baby poop. The WHO recommends exclusively breastfeeding (no food other than boobie milk) for the first six months of the little bubba's life. You see, human milk is a bit of a superhero, providing a host of benefits to mama and baby. However, a lot of people struggle with exclusively breastfeeding, and even though 'breast is best', this struggle can lead to a deep feeling of guilt in the mom. So, supplementing with additional infant formula or pumping breast milk is totally fine! In fact, there is a thriving market for human milk, and there are actual human milk banks where you can buy fresh boob juice. It gets even better. In 2011, for a very limited period, a London store sold an ice cream made of . . . wait for it . . . human breast milk called 'Baby Gaga' (excuse me while I die from laughing too hard). It was quickly put a stop to by the city authorities because of . . . concerns (LOL). Questionable ice cream aside, if you ever do start leaking milk from your breasts without any stimulation and you're not pregnant, you should see your doctor. This could be because of stress, infection, a hormonal imbalance, or even cancer. Your boobs should not be free milkshake dispensers unless there is a baby in the picture.

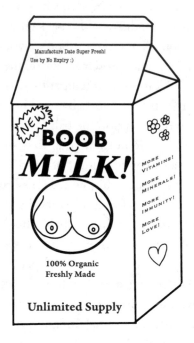

Speaking of babies and milkshakes, why the hell do men have nipples when they're not breastfeeding anyone? What is the purpose? Well, it turns out that nipples are the very first thing to develop in our bodies when we are embryos. As you've learnt in the chapter on clitoris (Chapter 6), the original blueprint of the human body is female. It's only under the influence of testosterone that a foetus starts developing as a male. Until then, it's exactly the same. And because nipples develop so early on, even before a foetus starts producing testosterone, men are left with nipples even though they don't need them. And while everyone has nipples, not everyone has breasts. Some men can develop boobies in a condition called gynaecomastia or man boobs. This results from a hormonal imbalance and leads to male boobs developing gland tissue, not fat. It can be caused by hormonal issues, certain medications, and even some drugs like marijuana. If you have sprouted unwanted boobs, it's a good idea to talk to your doctor, who can help treat the underlying issue and make your new boobies go away.

All in all, boobs are quite important in this galaxy. Hell, even the word 'galaxy' comes from the Greek word 'gala' meaning 'milk' because the ancients thought that the beautiful band of light that we can see around our Earth looks like milk. I mean, we live in something called the Milky Way galaxy (this one is quite obvious, so I'll let you come to this conclusion on your own). We seriously like boobies. Breasts have been loved, hated, vilified, and worshipped throughout world history. But breasts have also been greatly misunderstood. Mammals literally mean 'the one with breasts'. Boobs make us *us*. Everybody loves boobies: babies, old people, people who have them, people who don't have them; boobies are adored by one and all. And why shouldn't they be? Everyone has breasts no matter your gender, and all breasts are great breasts. And I hope you and your boobs become breast friends!

8

The Testicles

Listen, some men care way too much about their penis so I'm gonna start with the balls because the testicles are like, seriously important, and we don't pay them enough attention for some strange reason, except to make jokes that they hurt when you kick them. Don't believe me? Okay, tell me what do you know about the balls, other than the fact that they hurt when you kick them? See! I told you. Now, let me tell you about balls, and how they're related to avocados (seriously, I'm not joking).

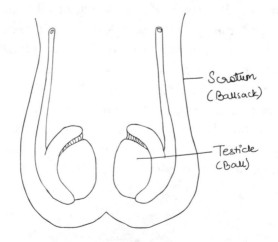

So . . . balls. They're called balls because they kinda look like . . . balls (lol), although they are more oval-shaped and the technical term is testicles or testes. Most people have two balls (Karan–Arjun type, they're both *bhai–bhai*) that hang inside a small pouch of skin in the crotch called a scrotum— aka ball sack, the little sack in which balls hang out—right behind the penis. Usually, one testicle hangs lower or is bigger than the other. More commonly, the right one is bigger, and the left one is lower hanging. Interestingly, an extensively researched study found that people who have lower hanging right testicles tend to be left-handed! Just like your penis, your balls grow in size too when you're turned on, almost by 50 per cent! Each testicle is about 2–3 inches long, and feels quite smooth . . . like an egg. I'm guessing that's probably how they get their Hindi name? Also, did you know that a common slang for testicles in Spanish is 'huevos', which also means eggs? This *anda* joke crosses geographic and linguistic barriers. Interestingly, the testicles themselves also look a bit like eggs. That's because the outermost layer of the testicles is made up of a tough shell that is grey-white in colour and is called the Tunica Albuginea, or White Tunic; it is smooth, like an egg. On the inside, however, it's a whole different convoluted story (literally). You remember those old-timey telephones that had a long coiled wire? Yeah, your testicles are full of something like that. Under the white tunic, testes have tubes that look like the coiley wire-like substance called seminiferous tubules, where sperm are produced. Essentially, your body makes sperm in something that looks like Maggi noodles inside your balls. And that, my friends, is the function of your testicles: they make sperm—and other things, but

sperm is pretty important for, y'know, us humans existing.
Along with this, our testicles also make hormones. Now most
glands, i.e., organs that make hormones, are actually internal,
or inside the body, but the testes are quite literally way too
cool for that. They hang outside the body in the pouch-
like scrotum. This is important because your testicles are
big fans of air-conditioning and work much better in cooler
environments.

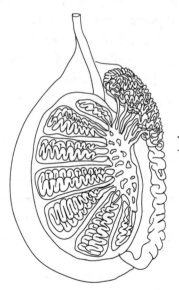

See!
I told you
the testicles are
full of noodles

In order to carry out this cool thing of temperature regulation,
your testes do another really cool thing of moving up and
down. The testicles are suspended in the scrotum by a cord
called the spermatic cord, which, along with some muscles,
can move your testicles in response to changes in temperature
so that your testicles are not getting fried (or frozen) from

your own body heat (or lack of it). This is also why your scrotum is all wrinkly like a raisin: it can provide more skin that way. So, when it's hot and sweaty, your testes stretch out all this wrinkly skin and hang the balls lower and further away from our body heat; and when it's cold, your scrotum shrinks and gets pulled up close to your body, keeping your balls nice and cosy. Interestingly, your body pulls your balls close to your body for safekeeping when it thinks you are in danger. Pretty cool, huh (literally)? Doing this is really important since the sperm factory inside your testes requires a constant temperature of around 35 degrees Celsius to make the best quality and quantity of sperm.

Remember that the testicles are actually inside the ball sack, and you only see the wrapper aka scrotum outside. Think of your scrotum as the furry jacket that protects your precious little kiddos. It's usually darker in colour than the rest of your skin, is wrinkly, and now we know why, and is covered in hair. It grows darker with puberty and that's a sign of sexual maturity; you absolutely do not need to lighten it. Some people might notice some lighter coloured bumps on the penis or scrotum (and on your lips and inner cheeks). These bumps are called Fordyce spots and are just oil glands that secrete a natural oil called sebum, which helps moisturize your skin. They usually become bigger at puberty, which is when you're more likely to notice them, but once again, this is completely natural. Stretching your skin, such as when you're having an erection, can make these more noticeable. Aside from the hairless parts, the scrotum is covered in pubic hair, which you will learn more about later.

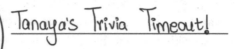

Tanaya's Trivia Timeout!

Normally, your oil glands are found around hair follicles, but in areas where there are fewer or no hair follicles, you end up seeing these glands. When on the genitals and cheeks, these are called Fordyce spots. Sometimes you might also see tiny bumps around your nipple called Tubercles of Montgomery. They're similar oil factories and nothing to worry about!

This pubic hair sprouts up when you hit puberty, somewhere around the age of 14. Your testicles grow, sometimes by as much as 500 per cent, and start producing hormones—which in turn make you grow taller, stronger, and grow body hair—and sperm, which you produce 24/7 until death! This sperm is endlessly produced inside your seminiferous tubules—up to a 100 million mature sperm per day—which can pair up with an egg and make a baby. Vitamin deficiencies, smoking, alcohol, injury to the testicles, and infectious diseases can all reduce how much sperm you make, so a healthy lifestyle means healthy little guys (ditch that cigarette bro). Anabolic steroids, you know, like the kind at the gym, can impact your sperm number and quality even up to the point of infertility, and also make your testes smaller. Heavy use of these steroids also come with other fun side effects like baldness, acne, erectile dysfunction, loss of libido, and even some cancers. Stay off those steroids, my dude. Your testicles also shrink in size with age, but that's just normal ageing and nothing to be worried about. With that being said, the size of your balls has nothing to do with how much sperm you make! Naturally small testicles make just as good sperm as naturally large testicles—size truly doesn't matter! (Unless you are a chimpanzee. Fun fact, chimpanzees have MASSIVE balls that make massive amounts of sperm all the time. This is because chimps love to bang: male and female chimps will have sex left, right, and centre. At any given time, a female chimp will have sperm in her from many male chimps; with so much competition, each chimp makes lots of sperm to increase its chances of becoming Chimp Daddy. Some strange data from some very strange research has shown that men who have larger balls have a higher likelihood of being cheaters, whereas men with smaller balls tend to become better fathers. I don't quite know what to make of that, so I will conveniently skip this and leave you to ponder.

But in order to make so much sperm, we need testosterone. But what is testosterone anyway? Testicles produce this hormone called testosterone and some other hormones, called androgens. Testosterone is the VIP of all androgens since it's essential for the development of 'male' reproductive organs like your dick and balls, and also facial hair, body hair, sex drive, muscles, and sperm. Women also make testosterone, and the testes are the male equivalent of ovaries, btw. (Testes ovaries twins *hain* basically.) It's at puberty when we start producing a lot of testosterone that we get *nayi nayi moonchein* and that newly developed deep voice.

Funnily though, ancient people also had some very strange beliefs about other things the testicles make. For example, some old-timey folks, such as the great Aristotle himself, believed that your right testicle made girl sperm and your left testicle made boy sperm. So the Ancient Greeks had this practice of cutting off their right testicle if they wanted to have boys. Obviously, that's bollocks but the weird stuff doesn't stop there: some cultures believe that eating animal testicles makes you more sexually potent and increases your penis size. The more culinarily adventurous among you are welcome to try and report back, although there is no scientific evidence that this works.

Since we are talking about testicles as food, I must inform you why I began this chapter mentioning the connection of testicles to avocados. Believe it or not, they are actually related: the Ancient Aztec word for avocados was ahuacatl, which means testicles. Probably because of what avocados look like when they are hanging from a tree, which gives a whole new meaning to 'creamy guacamole'. In more interesting stories about testicles and words, the word 'testify', which means providing evidence as a witness (like testifying in court) also comes from, you guessed it, testes! Apparently, in Ancient Rome, you would quite literally swear on your balls, holding your testicles, while making a public declaration of truth.

I told you. There's a lot more to balls than the fact that they hurt when you kick them.

9

The Penis

Okay, first off: it's not a 'pen-is'. It's a 'peenis'. If you want to be super medical, you can call it the intromittent organ (although nobody does and if you say that to a doctor, they'll probably think you're trying to pull a Shashi Tharoor and ignore you), or if you want to be chill, you can call it everything from dick, dong, nunnu, lingam, to more imaginative animal-oriented words like cock and anaconda. All of these words are talking about the same thing: this long organ that hangs between the legs and lets you do susu, bang, and brag about its size. Even though there is a lot to learn about this strange snake in your pants, we are somehow not able to

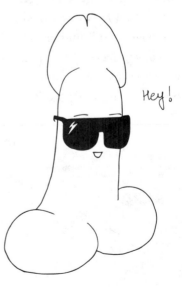

Hey!

move past how large or how small this organ should be. So, let's start by talking about Baby Penises. No, not like penises belonging to babies, but like tiny penises, when the penises were babies themselves, and their rise to greatness (pun very much intended).

A long, long time ago, when you were still a blueberry-sized little baby blob inside the uterus, there existed a tiny little mountain between your baby legs, called the genital bud. As we've learnt in Chapter 6, the penis and clitoris are *bhai–behen* and they originate from the same tissue aka the genital bud; this bud usually blossoms into a clitoris. But, if your building instructions are XY, i.e., genetically male, at some point around the second month, your blueberry-sized body grows teeny, tiny testicles that start making testosterone. This testosterone does some abracadabra shit and affects the clitoris, which grows bigger and bigger until it forms a penis. And ta-da! By week 14, when you're about the size of a kiwi, you have a penis and testicles! With your newly manufactured penis, you have by this point started to pee inside the uterus, which is making up a part of the amniotic fluid (baby juice) inside the amniotic sac (baby protective balloon).

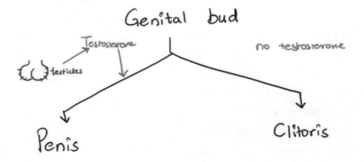

Genital bud

Testosterone

testicles

no testosterone

Penis

Clitoris

Now we have a fully functioning penis that is enthusiastically peeing away, which is one of the functions of the penis. The penis is connected to your bladder, pee storage bag, and all the collected pee made by your kidneys exits the body using this big gutter inside the penis, called the urethra. To understand this better, let's understand the structure of the penis.

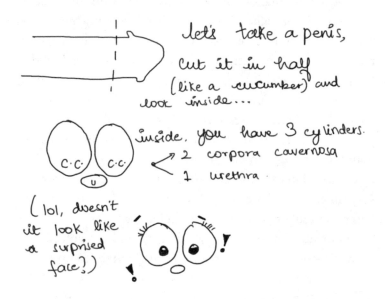

let's take a penis, cut it in half (like a cucumber) and look inside...

inside, you have 3 cylinders.
2 corpora cavernosa
1 urethra.

C.C. C.C.
U

(lol, doesn't it look like a surprised face?)

The penis is made up of three main structures—think of it like two *kathi* rolls and one straw. The straw pipe is your urethra, which helps you pee. The other two *kathi* roll pipes are important for doing some very hard work (I will stop with the penis jokes, I promise). These two *kathi* roll–like structures lie side-by-side and are called the corpora cavernosa or cave-like bodies. They are a bit like balloons, and can expand greatly in size and you probably know where I am going with this. Your penis is surrounded by blood vessels that expand when you're turned on and send a lot of blood into your penis to give you a strong erection. The same way as you can take a *kathi* roll and stuff it with paneer or chicken to make a bigger *kathi* roll, your body stuffs the penis *kathi* rolls with blood to make a big penis, aka cause an erection. You should know, smoking causes these blood vessels to become less elastic, allowing less blood to fill your *kathi* roll . . . err . . . penis. This is why smoking can be bad for your peepee. Once stuffed, the blood gets trapped inside, making your penis quite stiff, which, along with some help from your pelvic floor muscles, helps you maintain an erection and insert your penis into your orifice of choice. This fulfils the other role of your penis—to do sexy times, (and share your DNA with another human being and potentially make more human beings).

Human penises are significantly more evolved and sophisticated in their erection section, when compared to other animals. While we run this complex and cool blood-pumping party, other animals like dogs and gorillas have taken the easier evolutionary route and have a whole bone in their penis called a baculum. There are some seriously interesting interpretations regarding this penis bone correlated with the Adam and Eve and Eve emerging from Adam's rib story, and maybe you should go Google that now. Interestingly, even though humans don't have a penis bone, we can still fracture the penis. But more on that later.

Bone or no bone, a healthy penis is quite enthusiastic about erections. Some studies report that most men experience up to eleven erections a day, and two to five erections every night. You can even wake up with erections, very poetically called 'morning wood', which is normal. Penises like to stand to attention so much that doctors have even discovered erections in tiny babies inside the uterus. Obviously, you won't remember those intrauterine dick salutes because most people remember their first erections only from around the ages of twelve to fourteen, right after they hit puberty. Erections can come in a wide variety of shapes, curves, and directions—the penis can point upwards, downwards, sideways, or have a slight curve to it. These are all normal variations and nothing to be worried about. The one thing that does worry most people though is not the direction or curve. Most people tend to freak out about . . . bigness.

Let's talk about penis size! This is, ahem, a huge question. We put A LOT of pressure on men about the size of one particular body part, which is especially baffling because size really doesn't matter. That's right, you can have any size penis and it won't affect how much pleasure your partner feels—unless it's monstrously huge, in which case sex can be painful. You already know because you've read the clitoris chapter (and if not, why not?) that penetration does not lead to orgasms for most vulva owners. Yet, somehow, we are obsessed with anomalously large phalluses. Look through the DMs of any of your female friends; I'm sure you'll find at least one text boasting about a 12-inch penis expecting them to be impressed by that. Penises under 2.5 inches, when it is officially classified as a micro penis, are found in less than

0.6 per cent of the population. And even then, people with a micro penis can have pleasurable sex and have children!

Now, if yours is over 2.5 inches and you are wondering what the average size of an erect penis is, you'd be surprised to learn that it's not as horse-sized as porn seems to suggest. In fact, most studies place an average erect penis between 5.1 inches to 5.5 inches. Solidly under what porn wants you to believe. No, seriously, research has shown that over 85 per cent of men overestimate the size of an average penis and feel insecure about their own penis size. This impacts their confidence, relationships, sexual life, and sense of satisfaction with their own body, which can all lead to stress and anxiety. And what do stress and anxiety do? Stress releases chemicals in your body that make your blood vessels smaller, restricting the amount of blood reaching your penis, making your perfectly normal-sized healthy penis unable to have an erection. Stress is a very real cause of erectile dysfunction. And if you smoke when you're stressed, it compounds the problem even further.

So, screw penis size. It doesn't matter, and an average penis is smaller than you'd think. But is that a bad thing? Are small penises bad? Do they affect how much pleasure your partner feels? Are colossal penises important for your partner to have an orgasm? What is this size-related pleasure dicktatorship? Once again, I am here to remind you, SIZE DOES NOT MATTER. And why? Because penetration ≠ orgasms. There is no magic orgasm button deep inside the vagina or anus that will make your partner instantly orgasm. It doesn't matter if the pole you're using to scratch your back is long or short if the itch is on your arm. Go back to the clitoris.

With that said, there are some actual things that do affect your penis size: hormones, body fat, injury, and age. So, penis size is determined when you're inside the uterus, and is influenced by a 'cock'tail of hormones called 'androgens', of which testosterone is the most important. During certain periods of your life, such as childhood and puberty, testosterone is really important in determining the size of your future penis. If a deficiency is recognized at this stage, well and good; you can treat it using hormones. However, taking testosterone post puberty has nooo effect on your penis size. No need to look up testosterone injections on the dark web; so you can close your browser now. Other factors that can impact your penis include injury, which can cause your penis to change shape due to scar tissue being formed, shortening the length or making it more curved, and age as reduced blood flow over a long period of time can cause penis atrophy. Seriously, ditch those cigarettes and monitor your cholesterol. Now, people who have lost a lot of weight will swear to you that losing weight makes your dick bigger. While losing *excess* body fat can be good for your health in many different ways, it doesn't actually make your penis bigger . . . it just makes the penis *appear* bigger. You see, the penis can be hidden due to a fat pouch, especially in the belly area. Morbid obesity can cause the penis to be almost buried in fat of the surrounding tissue, making it look stubbier than it is. Obviously, losing weight doesn't make your penis actually change size, just as losing weight doesn't make your foot smaller. It only causes an apparent change in length—like an optical illusion, just like the 'objects in the mirror might be closer than they appear' warning on your car *ka* side mirror. Want an easier fix to make your penis look bigger, other than losing a couple of kilos? Trim the surrounding bush! Although, again, that just makes it *appear* larger, and shaving your pubes comes with its own set of risks.

Small, medium, large, XL, no matter what size penis you have, all our penises are born with a special sweater. A turtleneck, if you will. This extra layer of skin that sits atop the penis like a scarf is called the foreskin. You can move this around, pull it back and forth, and it is fairly stretchy. On the inner side, the surface is like the inside of your mouth (there are some oral sex jokes here that I'm too lazy to make). The foreskin does two main jobs: provides some lubrication (yes, penises need lube too) and protects the penis, especially in childhood, when your peepee is often sitting in a diaper full of pee and poop. Considered to be the oldest planned surgery in the world, some religions and cultures have this practice of surgically removing the foreskin, called circumcision; some medical conditions also require this surgery. Now, this is a hotly contested topic in science: we have research that suggests that in *high-risk populations*, circumcised people have lower rates of HIV and other STIs, especially in Sub-Saharan Africa, but any advantages of this procedure in the nonhigh-risk populations are kinda meh. We also have some evidence from Sub-Saharan Africa that circumcised people have a reduced risk of contracting human papillomavirus (HPV), urinary tract infections (UTIs), and certain types of cancer. However, there are *many* questions about the ethics of this practice: you see, circumcision is performed mostly on babies who are too young to understand the process and give consent. If done consensually, the WHO actually recommends circumcision for adults in areas that have high levels of HIV infections. All medical institutions, at the end of the day, do believe that if done, this procedure must be carried out by trained professionals. Not by some rando wielding a knife near your, ahem, special parts. If done by untrained hands, this process can also go horribly wrong causing catastrophic bleeding, infections, and injury to the penis. Let's leave this one to the experts, shall we?

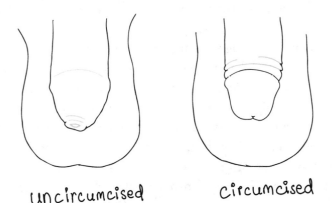

uncircumcised   circumcised

Other than taking off this special penis sweater, there are some *very* interesting beautification procedures performed on the penis. Just like the vulva, our dear penis friend also has some unrealistic beauty standards to uphold all across the globe. Foreskin or penis piercing, penis tattooing, or even inserting small beads under the surface of the penis are all done to enhance sensitivity. From Borneo, we have the especially painful technique of *ampallang*, where a genital piercing goes through the entire head of the penis. This has the fun side effect of being rather difficult to heal, and also causing tooth injuries to your partner when receiving oral sex from them. From Japan, we have the bizarrely adorable tradition of cock + origami = *kokigami*, which is the art of making costumes for the penis out of folded paper. This strange rendition of penile Halloween is a very ancient practice, and claims to enhance sexual pleasure. Maybe that's something you'll just have to try out for yourself? Aside from these rather questionable beautification procedures, we also have a very long cultural love affair with the penis.

Many years ago, while travelling through Bhutan, my mother and I were very surprised to see giant penises everywhere—on doorways, walls, signs, hanging in cars, paintings, sculptures—every form of penis art decorates the ancient, quiet country of Bhutan. They even worship it! Pompeii, the ancient Roman city destroyed by a volcanic eruption, is one of the most fascinating sights in the world. The ash from the eruption buried the whole city, perfectly preserving it for close to 2000 years. Centuries later, when it was rediscovered, historians were surprised to find GIANT PENISES everywhere! Apparently, they were supposed to be (extremely suggestive) arrows pointing you in the direction of the nearest brothel. We've loved the penis throughout history, you guys. Unlike the clitoris, there is a lot of study and research on the penis. Why, there is even a massive museum in Iceland dedicated entirely to penises. The Phallological Museum in Iceland houses everything from the tiny baculum (penis bone) of a hamster, visible only with a magnifying glass, all the way to a giant 67-inch *tip* of a blue whale penis. (Yes, only the tip. Blue whale penises are, on average, as large as 10 feet long).

Penis research is pretty intense. In fact, a bird researcher at Yale University managed to secure close to $500,000 for studying duck penises. For good reason though—duck penises are crazy cool! They are corkscrew-shaped and MASSIVE. Like the length of their entire body massive (imagine a human penis the size of a human being; sorry for the nightmares). Donald Dick, uh sorry, Donald Duck is starting to look very different now, isn't he? Okay, now that we have reached this point, I must tell you more. Ducks are some of the only birds in the animal kingdom to have a penis at all; most birds boink by touching their special parts together in a process called the cloacal kiss. This corkscrew-shaped nightmare also goes from zero to fully erect in one-third of a second, beating any supercar you know. I know you did not pick this book up expecting to know about duck penises in such detail, but this stuff is too incredible to not share. Basically, everything about duck penises is interesting, as a great article is titled on Jezebel. And I'm going to use duck dicks to segue into lizard dicks to close this chapter and end it with this incredible joke I read.

'Why didn't the lizard have a girlfriend?'
'Cuz he had a reptile dysfunction.'

Lol.

10

Pubic Hair

I'm 99.99 per cent sure that you have either already removed or tried to remove your pubic hair at some point in your life— by shaving, waxing, trimming, using hair removal creams, plucking every single hair out one-by-one. Okay I don't think anyone has ever done that last one.

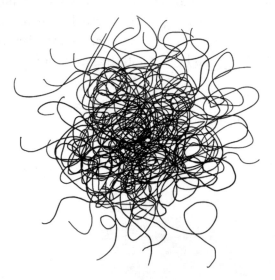

So, why does pubic hair exist? Does it serve a purpose? And is it important to remove your pubes? You know how in old-timey fairy tales there is always a dense and dangerous forest that the prince needs to cross in order to go kiss his princess inside the palace? Yeah, your pubes are like that—they act as a dense forest that exists outside the palace of your 'private parts', guarding and protecting them. Your pubes are good for you—they protect the sensitive skin of your genitals from irritation, act as a very hairy cushion to reduce the friction we experience during sex, trap any dirt and bad bugs that might be harmful, add humidity so that your skin feels moist, and even act like a little sweater to keep your genitals nice and warm! Not only that, your pubes may also function as a status update to other people to let them know you are available for sexy times. Thousands of years ago, back in the time when we lived like the Flintstones, your pubes would be an important indicator to others that you've gone through puberty, and are ready to do Yabba Dabba Doo and make babies! Some scientists also believe that pubic hair plays an important role in helping spread your 'pheromones', which are basically sexy-time chemicals produced by your body. The hair acts like a trap, so your genitals can keep smelling all sexy and pheromone-y, and any potential partner will know that you are down to party all night. We don't really know if they do this, or even if pheromones exist, but this is one of the theories!

This hair forest is pretty dense and lush, and even if you have straight hair on the top of your head, pubic hair is usually curly for most people. You have your hormones *ka kamaal* to thank for this *kaale, lambe, ghane baal* situation.

As you hit puberty, the level of testosterone in your body rises, which makes hair grow and you beautifully start resembling our ape cousins. This also causes hair to grow in your armpits, around your butthole, and all around your body. Pubic hair covers the genitals and often extends up to the inner thighs and up to the tummy. While the idea can be very entertaining, you cannot actually make *chotis* out of your pubic hair, as pubes are slightly different from the hair on your head and do not grow indefinitely. Pubic hair also doesn't have to match the hair colour on your head and can, in fact, come in a variety of colours. It even greys as we grow older!

With this puberty purchase of pubic hair, you get a free offering of more sebaceous glands in these areas that secrete oil, called sebum, to keep your skin moist. This sebum, plus special sweat glands coupled with the resident bacteria of our skin, give the very nice, distinctive smell that we associate with our pubes, and our pubic hair helps these smells reach far and wide!

Actually, this stuff is really interesting; these special sweat glands deserve more attention! So, we have two kinds of sweat glands: eccrine glands, which secrete the thin and smell-free sweat that keeps you cool when you're getting hot; and apocrine glands in your genitals and armpits, which release a delicious, fatty kind of sweat (dude, fat is delicious) that our skin bacteria love to feed on. The smell in our sweat is pretty much from these bacteria; it results from the digestion and breakdown of this fatty sweat. So, *you* probably don't smell, you just have enthusiastically farty bacteria on you!

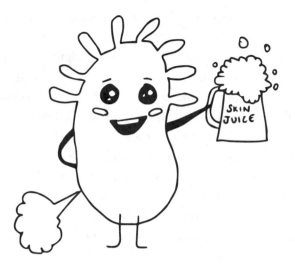

Getting rid of your pubic hair obviously reduces the general genital-y smell in your genitals. Removing the hair reduces the amount of surface area or space for bacteria to stick on and grow, which means the bacteria become homeless and don't have their oil-rich food anymore and cannot fart away to glory. But this does not mean that having pubic hair is dirty. These bacteria live on our hair AND our skin and are not bad for us. In fact, our farty friends are really important for us to maintain healthy skin. Removing pubic hair just reduces the intensity of our natural smell. But people still like to remove their pubic hair for many reasons, and if you want to remove your hair, you do you, boo! I just want to have a chat—because I don't think we really get to schedule a consult with our doctors about how to effectively manage our bush—about how to do it in the most safe way, if you have to . . . and if you actually *need* to remove this hair.

Let's begin with this thought: in all the porn, medical images, art, dolls, media depictions, descriptions, conversations, how often have you seen pubes? Barely ever, right? We've been very energetic about de-pubing ourselves throughout human history. Apparently, some of the oldest rituals of pubic hair removal come from India from as early as 5000 years ago (but I haven't found a very reliable source for this claim so we will take this with a grain of salt)! Genital hair is so systematically removed from public discourse that a lot of people find their bodies repulsive when they start sprouting this very natural hair. The prevalence of baby butt-ly smooth genitals is so profound that, in fact, John Ruskin, a very famous Western art critic, was horrified on his wedding night when he saw an actual naked woman for the first time, as opposed to the more, ahem, stylized and hair-free depictions in art. On seeing his new bride's magnificent bush, he thought she was deformed and HE RAN AWAY. He ran away because he thought his wife was a monster for having pubic hair. You might think that such a hysterically hilarious (and sad) thing would never happen in today's world, but I will remind you of the question we began this paragraph with: How often have you seen pubic hair in film, media, art, or mainstream porn? I wouldn't be surprised if something like this happens in today's day and age either.

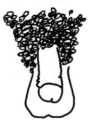

But trends come and go, and just as it's historically been fashionable to be completely bald like a *taklu* downstairs, it has also been fashionable to grow a lush garden between your legs. The Ancient Indians and Egyptians were said to be fans of copper razors, and the Greeks and Romans considered no pubic hair as the ideal. Even the *Kama Sutra* says that 'a man about town' should have all his body hair removed every fifth or tenth day. This changed in the Middle Ages, when a full bush was preferred, and pubic hair removal was considered a symbol of prostitution. Diseases were rampant and pubic hair was (correctly) believed to protect from infections. Some people even shaved their pubic hair and then put on pubic hair wigs to hide the sores from diseases like syphilis and gonorrhoea. This took a turn during the Renaissance era when pubes went out of fashion again. One of the most popular methods of getting rid of pubic hair was by using a sort of an old-world hair-removal cream, where people would apply a mix of arsenic (yes, arsenic) and quicklime to the skin, taking care to wash off the mixture before it burnt their skin.

The real game changer in our story was a popular razor manufacturer. He wanted to increase profits from his razor sales, and so he thought of creating a new market and doubling his clientele: In 1915, the women's razor was born. Razors were still considered super masculine, so he came up with some pretty nifty tricks, which are still in use in advertising to this day, to make women's razors popular. He added shame and insecurity. Gillette ads would say things like 'solve an embarrassing personal problem' about body hair, implying that body hair was a problem and embarrassing. The shady marketing stuck, and we continue to believe pubic hair is bad and needs to be removed.

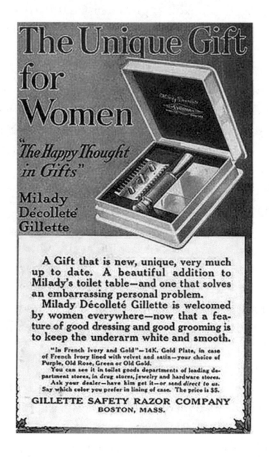

This is untrue. Pubic hair is meant to protect you. It is not dirty or disgusting. It's just hair! However, if you still want to get rid of your pubic hair, do it in the correct way. I don't recommend waxing the pubes as it can lead to burns and irritation. Getting your pubes lasered off is fine, but it doesn't work for everyone. If you opt or it, make sure you get this done by a trained professional or you could get pretty severe burns. Because of the risk of burns, as your genital skin is more sensitive, I strictly advise against the use of hair removal creams on your pubic hair. Just don't. And if you're going to shave, always use a fresh razor (and no, shaving does not make your hair grow back thicker). Shave in the direction of hair growth; this will help in preventing ingrown hair, which can lead to those small boils you might see on your genitals after you shave. Please, take care. The injuries from pubic hair removal can get seriously infected. Some doctors especially recommend that diabetics not remove their pubes, because it increases risk of an infection. We also have some data to show that removing your pubic hair increases your risk of STIs. Having pubic hair not only reduces your risk of STIs by acting as a barrier, but also helps keep your skin moist. If you experience a lot of dryness on your vulva, stop removing your pubes. If you still experience a lot of dryness, applying soothing natural oils like olive oil can help. Either way, it's your body, so make the best possible decisions for yourself, by yourself. Nobody gets to tell you what to do with your own body.

Universally loved, hated, fetishized, collected (yes, that too!)—our pubes have a very interesting history. But maybe, it's time we also gave them some respect and just left them the hell alone. After all, love is in the hair.

Ew! What's That Goo?!

11

Semen

The internet is full of some very strange things. For example, did you know that you can buy a delightfully titled book called *Natural Harvest*, which details many different and might I say, ingenious, ways you can cook with semen. The back cover is . . . very interesting, claiming, 'Like fine wine and cheeses, the taste of semen is complex and dynamic. Semen is inexpensive to produce and is commonly available in many, if not most, homes and restaurants.' If that's not intriguing enough for you, you can also look for *Semenology: The Semen Bartender's Handbook*, which promises to teach you how to 'mix selected spirits to enhance the delicate flavour of semen' and 'add a personal touch to any cocktail'. Truly personal, indeed.

But is there any truth to these books or are they just gag gifts (in more ways than one)? What is semen? How is it different from sperm? And are there really any nutritional benefits to consuming it, or is it just a load of jizz? Is it vegan-friendly (I aim to be asking the most important science questions, after all)? What's the deal with spitting versus swallowing? Why does it taste so icky? Why is it so sticky (rhyme!)? And why on earth does it have such a funky smell? So, let's cum on (sorry) and drown ourselves (sorry again) in semen knowledge.

Semen is the white gunk that shoots out from a penis on ejaculation. While an average ejaculate is only half a teaspoon, it contains a lot. A lot, lot, lot. Literally, millions of sperm. Okay wait, I'm getting ahead of myself. Let's go back to the start. So, semen is made up of two main parts: seminal fluid (95 per cent) and sperm (5 per cent); yes, semen and sperm are two different things. Sperm makes up a surprisingly small part of semen, but it is super powerful as it's responsible for the continued existence of our species (and several other species) across the planet. That's because sperm contains half of the secret to life, the very building blocks, the blueprint of human life; sperm contains DNA. These microscopically tiny, tadpole-shaped, DNA-containing little wiggling bits club with the other half of your building block DNA (from your mom) to make *you*. Not only that, but the sex of the baby is determined by the sperm; you see, while eggs are *always* girl eggs (XX), with sperm we can have boy sperm (XY) and girl sperm (XX). So, girl egg + girl sperm, makes a girl, duh. But a girl egg + boy sperm will make a boy. Depending on which sperm is fertilizing the egg, the future sex of the baby is decided. But in order to make the long, perilous, fertilization journey, from inside the testicles, out through the penis, into the vagina, past the cervix, up into the uterus, all the way into the Fallopian tubes, where it will meet the egg (wow that is long indeed, especially for something so tiny) the sperm needs energy, and lots of it. Thankfully, sperm comes floating in its own energy drink!

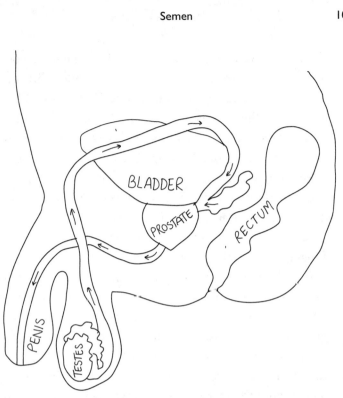

This energy drink, which is semen, contains everything the sperm needs for surviving its long journey. Think of it like a milkshake made of juices from different places across the reproductive tract. To make this semen milkshake at home, you will need juices from the seminal vesicles, the prostate, and the bulbourethral glands (BUG). The seminal vesicles make this fructose (sugar) rich juice, which makes up 70–80 per cent of semen and helps provide energy to the sperm to swim. Think of it like *ganne ka* juice (sugarcane juice) for sperm. To this, add a squeeze of clear-white fluid from the prostate. This contains enzymes, micronutrients, and fat. Think of it like the milk of your milkshake. Now add some ooey gooey mucus-y fluid from the BUG. They will help add lubrication to your semen milkshake, and help it slide down easily. BUGs make pre-cum. Pre-cum is the clear fluid that can leak out of the penis before ejaculation. It also helps make your urethra (peeing and cumming pipe) less acidic from whatever leftover urine there might be, to allow sperm to survive. To this, add some essential micronutrients, some amines, some more weird complex sounding chemicals, about 50–200 million sperm, and you have . . . a teaspoon of semen!

This teaspoon of semen is highly alkaline, to buffer the acidic pH of the vagina as otherwise the acidity of the vagina will kill all the sperm. It also contains some secretions from the prostate that make it thick and gooey so that it is again protected from the villainous vagina. This extra dose of prostatic goo eventually dissolves away in a process called liquefaction, which occurs around thirty minutes after ejaculation, once the sperm have gone well beyond the vagina. This is why it's easier to clean jizz off of you right after an orgasm. If you leave it sitting there for a while, it will become a liquid-y, runny messy, all thanks to the prostate secretions. Also, did you know, some studies have found that regular ejaculations reduce your risk of prostate cancer? (The prostate is a small, walnut-sized gland inside the body. It's also called the 'male G-spot' as some people can have an orgasm from directly stroking it. You can reach the prostate by sticking your finger inside your butt, and stroking the front wall gently. It has a notorious reputation for, *aise hi free fund mein*, growing really fat in old age, which can cause problems with peeing in older men. It's also a very common site for cancer.

So, fap away to glory, my friends, and protect yourself from a common cancer.

All this sounds really really good. Semen sounds like it's got a lot of fantastic nutritional benefits. So, should we go around swallowing it? Well, as we've learnt, semen does contain fructose, protein, citric acid, sugar, zinc, lots of vitamins (especially B and C), and many other essential nutrients; but not in enough quantities to make it nutritionally relevant. It's super low calorie though. And thanks to various amines in semen, like cadaverine and putrescine (the compounds that give rotting flesh its smell), it can have a very distinct odour. So, you can swallow if you like, but there are no 'benefits' of swallowing it. It can come with risks though, since unprotected oral sex comes with the disadvantage of exposing you to STIs. So, if you have *any* unprotected oral sex, you are exposed to the risk of STIs, whether or not you swallow. Swallowing does not add any additional dangers. If you want to avoid these dangers, but still enjoy oral sex, always remember to use dental dams and condoms. Do what you will with that and your delicate palate.

A curious study (like your curious palate) has (questionably) shown that sperm may have some antidepressant properties. Researchers followed college-going women, and found that women who used condoms when having sex had higher rates of depression and suicidal attempts compared with women who did not. This sounds like a very good case of causation versus correlation to me, which basically means that just because two things are related does not mean one causes the other. For example, people like to eat a lot of mithai around Diwali. Around this time of the year, there is also an increase in firecracker-related injuries. So, one could hypothesize that mithai causes firecracker injuries. But this makes no sense, right? Just because two random events occur around the same time doesn't necessarily mean they cause each other. And that, my friends, is causation versus correlation. And so, I will ask you to take this study with a grain of salt (or a drop of salty water, teehee). Keep using those condoms.

Other than spitting or swallowing, or making babies, there are some more interesting ways to . . . ahem, use semen. Some people enjoy ejaculating on another person's face, which is called a 'facial'. Facials have the (dubious) honour of being the most popular type of external ejaculation, featuring in almost 62 per cent of all porn videos showing someone cumming on someone else. Some studies have shown that up to 96 per cent of all of the bestselling heterosexual porn has shown a man gloriously cumming on a woman's body. Critics and gender researchers have raised questions about this as, a lot of times this can be a part of subjugating and humiliating their female partners, with no regard for what the woman wants. It's great if you and your partner enjoy it, but please do not coerce your partner into doing this. It can be very violent, traumatic, and humiliating.

Not only can it be demeaning, but it can also go catastrophically wrong, as some people can be allergic to semen. Um, yes. A literal allergic reaction in which there is a super rare allergy against the proteins in semen. It has been observed almost exclusively in women, where they notice redness, itching, burning, swelling, and hives on areas that come in contact with semen. There can be swelling on the tongue and throat, shortness of breathing, nausea, vomiting, and just a crap load of illness after a jizzload. The treatment, aside from using condoms and pre-sex anti allergic medications, is . . . sex. I mean, not exactly. The treatment involves a doctor exposing the vagina to extremely diluted semen over a long period of time. Once the treatment is 'over', the couple must have sex often, at least once every forty-eight hours, or the allergy could return. Talk about having an itch.

Now obviously, that semen-diluting doctor has a very um, interesting job. But did you know that there are actual semen doctors out there? Like they're dedicated to being doctors of semen, the semen-making process, and the semen-making apparatus. These guys are called andrologists, and one of the ways they check whether your semen is healthy or not is by doing a test called semen analysis. In a semen analysis, andrologists check for things like the amount, colour, viscosity (how thicc your jizz is), and the pH of your semen, plus the number, type, look, and concentration of sperm in your semen. Normally, you produce between 2–5 ml (a teaspoon-ish) of grey-white, alkaline semen containing between 50–200 million sperm.

If something weird comes up, andrologists can treat it with medications, and repeat the test in two to three months. This is because your sperm-making factory gets a reset and delivers a fresh new batch every 72-ish days. I mean, you keep making sperm from puberty to death, so quality inspections and improvements are very important, after all. (So, if you're planning to or trying to have a baby, give yourself at least two months and quit all the *sutta* and bad stuff. And then try properly with a fresh, A1-quality sperm delivery. A good healthy diet, exercise, and stress-free environments are also recommended for a good sperm count. Obesity and physical inactivity, along with smoking, are some of the worst things you can do for your sperm.) Nowadays, you can also get some neat at-home semen analysis kits, that have a little attachment that slides into your phone and does an automated sperm count reading using your phone camera. Obviously, this test is not as detailed, but boy oh boy, the future has truly arrived. No wait. The future has cum (sorry not sorry).

Aside from the future cumming, you can also cum. Accidentally. In your sleep. I'm talking about nightfall, wet dreams, or 'nocturnal emissions', where you jizz your pants out of sheer night-time orgasmic delight. You don't have to be masturbating for this, and they're a common aspect of normal sexual development. They start around puberty, and everyone can have them for the rest of their life. They don't indicate any underlying problems and are just free orgasms (and who doesn't like free orgasms, you tell me?). Some studies have noticed that people who avoid masturbation have an increased chance of experiencing nocturnal emissions, but we don't know this for sure. This, of course, can pose a huge problem for people who don't want to have an orgasm. But wait, didn't we read that orgasms are good for you, and even protect you from cancer? Also, aren't they hella fun? So why wouldn't someone want to have an orgasm, solo or partnered?

And so, let me take you into a truly weird corner of the dudebro internet. There is a group of people who practice NoFap—a website and community that describes itself as a community-based *porn* recovery site—where they avoid watching porn and masturbating. They believe (correctly) that porn can be damaging for the brain. But they also believe (incorrectly) that masturbation or sometimes even having orgasms is bad for you. Angry (and confused) no-fappers fiercely proselytize, spreading their seed (lol) of anti-masturbatory thoughts far and wide. These ideas, coupled with some ancient, pseudo-scientific thoughts about the *supposed* ills of masturbation (such as hair loss, protein loss, blindness, hairy palms, what have you) plague the internet. They claim that not masturbating increases your testosterone levels, increases muscle growth, and cures erectile dysfunction. But then, what will you do with this extra testosterone, my dude?

Is there any research to back the wild claims made by them, or is it a jizzaster, as eminent urologist Dr Andrew Spitz very poetically puts it? Well . . . no. We don't have any good science to back up these claims. While there is no doubt that porn can be damaging for your brain, experts say that as long as sexual behaviour is not compulsive, it is okay and completely normal. Hell, masturbation isn't even a recognized addiction in medical science. Unfortunately, the myths are so strongly semented, uh sorry, cemented in the no-fapper heads that no amount of logic or science gets past. Interestingly, no-fap communities have been found to have ties to the anti-feminist movement, far-right ideologies, and reportedly have a lower trust in science too (yeah, no shit). These communities are also rife with misogyny. To add to that, the community is also very trigger happy about suing scientists who pursue masturbation research, filing court cases against sex researchers left, right, and centre.

I appreciate the original intent of the no-fap movement: porn can be very damaging and often lead to violent and compulsive behaviours. But is masturbation the devil's dance?

That's a very reductive and naive thought. We have the best medical research in the world to show that masturbation is a healthy practice that can have many benefits (detailed in a later chapter) and can be a great way of expressing self-love. And masturbation is different from semen retention.

Wait, what the duck is semen retention now? So, semen retention is an ancient practice across many different religions that basically says, enjoy sex but don't jizz, bro. It's also called 'coitus reservatus' and can also include dry orgasms (where you have an orgasm but don't ejaculate). This involves a lot of practice and serious pelvic floor control. A number of ancient practices and religions believe that semen is sacred and full of life force. But ancient people (the great Aristotle included) also thought that the max amount of sperm is in your head, between your eyes, so make of that scientific semen 'knowledge' what you will. These ideas were born in a time when it was believed that women have no contribution to reproduction, and all the baby-making happens only because of semen. There are no proven scientific benefits to semen retention, so if having an orgasm makes you happy, do it. If not having an orgasm makes you happy, also do it. But please don't believe that semen has some magical properties and keeping it stored inside you will make you a superhero.

Semen is so revered for its magical benefits (but vaginal discharge is dirty, uh-huh?) that some tribes in Papua New Guinea even believe that drinking semen (with a cursory blow job, of course) or 'male milk' is essential to grow up into a strong, masculine man. Young boys from these tribes, who haven't even achieved puberty, are first separated from their mothers, beaten, have sticks inserted in their nostrils to make them bleed (to build their pain tolerance), and then, well then, they're made to suck dick. And then swallow. It is believed that blowing and swallowing this precious man milk will make these young boys grow into big, strong warriors. Thankfully, there has been a sexual (and gender) revolution in these areas, along with some sex education, finally putting some of these harmful practices to rest. Semen contains DNA from your biological dad, not magic.

And once again, we come back to the eternal question that plagues (wo)mankind: to swallow or not to swallow. Well, the choice is entirely yours. Just make sure you're staying protected from sexually transmitted infections. And while semen has no nutritional or health benefits, some people do like ingesting semen—via cookbooks or ritualized homosexuality. Either way, bon appétit!

12

Periods

The very first person to say 'period' on a TV advert was Courtney Cox, the actress who played the iconic Monica Geller on the hit sitcom *Friends*. This was in 1985. Let that sink in. Up until 1985, which was just over 35 years ago, nobody had ever said 'period' on TV. That's how taboo periods have been. Actually, wait, it gets even more bizarre. The word 'taboo' comes from the Polynesian word 'tapu', which means 'forbidden' and is used to refer to periods in a sideways, wink-wink, nudge-nudge fashion. TABOO = PERIODS! What the bloody hell.

We haven't exactly been kind to periods, (and periods haven't been kind to us either, lol) throughout human history. The famous Roman dude Pliny the Elder had some pretty interesting views about periods 2000 years ago. He believed menstruating women would make land barren, dogs go mad, dull weapons just by looking at them, control the weather (hang on, this sounds hella powerful), and make wine go bad by touching it. The good people of mediaeval Europe thought period cramps were the divine punishment that women bear for Eve's original sin and, therefore, should not get any treatment for. They did have one very strange remedy though: Apparently, if you burn a toad and wear its ashes around your neck, your period pain will be gone. How you're going to get a toad and burn it is anyone's guess. Some ancient people thought period blood caused leprosy and some, on the other hand, thought it cured leprosy. Texts from ancient Egypt show that menstrual blood was used in ointments that claimed to prevent boobs from sagging. Texts and videos from modern social media show menstrual blood being used in facials for a youthful glow (don't do this, please). We've had a bloody complicated relationship with our periods. But what the hell are periods? What causes periods? What are normal periods? How often should you have periods? What about all the taboos around periods? Love them or hate them, you really can't ignore them. So, why not learn about our periods?

For most of history, we have had no idea about why periods exist and what they do. Up until 1831, barely 200 years ago, we had NO idea that periods were linked to ovulation and fertility. Before that, everyone thought periods were a way of detoxing your body, although why only people with a uterus were considered toxic enough to require a monthly detox? Smells like good ol' fashioned patriarchy. Eventually though, we did learn that periods are linked with your uterus being an old grandma who always wants a baby. If that sounds ridiculous, let me introduce to you how periods work with a story, of course.

Our story begins at menarche, the time when you start having your periods. Most people start this between nine and sixteen years of age. This is an exciting time in your life, full of changes in your body, thanks to all kinds of hormonal *lochebaazi*. When you're riding the puberty roller coaster, many new things start sprouting in the body like boobs and body hair, and blood starts coming out from your vagina every month. In the first one or two years, this blood waterfall isn't always regular and may not occur every month. But within a few months to a year, your uterus decides that it must squeeze itself every single month like a lemon and give your vagina a blood-bath. You'll find that your body sets into a pattern, and a regular period comes anytime between every twenty-one and forty days. This pattern can take up to two years to establish itself after you start period-ing. After that, if you get periods earlier than every 20 days or later than every 40 days, you should speak to your doctor. A normal period lasts anywhere between two to seven days, where you pass about two or three tablespoons of blood and mucus. You can experience bloating, tenderness in the breasts, acne, mood swings, and cramping pain in your tummy, lower back, and your legs right before or during your periods. Please note that severe pain or severe mood swings are not normal and worth getting investigated. If you track your cycles by noting down the date of your period and the common symptoms you experience, you will be able to identify what is normal for you. If you experience anything outside of your normal, you can always see your doctor, who can figure out if something is out of the ordinary.

How periods work isn't rocket science. (Although, we actually reached the moon before we started putting that sticky stuff on the back of the sanitary pad. Seriously. The adhesive strip on the back of the pad that helps hold it in place was added in 1969. The same year we sent a human being to the literal moon. We managed to send human beings into space before we could design a pad that stays put without moving around too much.)

But, periods are a fairly simple *kahaani*.

Think of your ovaries like a very serious school for high-performing kids. The ovary is full of kids, i.e., your eggs which want to study and go out and make the best damn career, i.e., babies in the world. So, your brain, the *head*master, (cuz it's inside the head. Gettit? Hehehe) sends some incredibly hardworking teachers (hormones) to your ovary school to instruct the students (eggs). Under the influence of hormones from the brain, the ovary develops lots of eggs. But Student of the Year . . . errr, sorry, month, is only one. So, while there are many student eggs studying in the ovary school, only one egg becomes the best, biggest, brightest egg. *Out of all the oocytes that develop, one egg becomes the main or the primary oocyte.* This is an ambitious student egg that wants to go out of the confines of its ovary school step out into the real world, and make a fantastic career (baby). So, this Smart Egg starts preparing to leave its ovary world behind, in a process called ovulation.

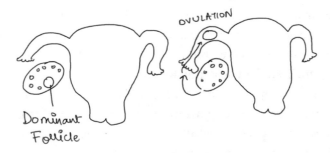

This cycle happens every month, so your body knows the drill. It knows that Smart Egg will soon leave this Ovary School and go off to university, i.e., uterus so they can fulfil their career dreams (make a baby). To achieve this, Smart Egg will need some support at their new university. And so, the body starts preparing a new home for this Smart Egg and their career at Uterus University. The body starts to build a cosy room, full of blankets, so Smart Egg can study well and work. *Under the influence of hormones, your body is building up a thick endometrium, (inside lining of the uterus) for a future baby that will develop when the egg meets a sperm.* Unfortunately, one more thing is super important for Smart Egg to be able to have their dream career: they need a scholarship, i.e., sperm. Without this sperm scholarship, Smart Egg will not have the sufficient means to have a thriving career and make a baby.

So, while the Smart Egg is still in school, the body already starts collecting many blankets to make the Uterus University room warm and comfortable. At some point, Smart Egg finally leaves Ovary School and starts looking for a scholarship on the way. If Egg can find a sperm scholarship, then they can reach Uterus University. *If after ovulation, egg and sperm meet, then fertilization happens. An embryo is formed, which goes into the uterus and gets implanted.* But if Egg is not able to secure this extra funding, the plans of the Uterus University fail, and there are tears of blood. Once Uterus University learns that their student will not be able to make it to study this semester, they start emptying out the room. All the lovely, plush blankets, (endometrium) that were collected are thrown out to make space, hopefully, for a new student next semester. *After ovulation, if the egg doesn't meet a sperm, the egg dies, and the uterus sheds off its inside lining in a menstrual period to prepare for next month.*

And that's how a period works!

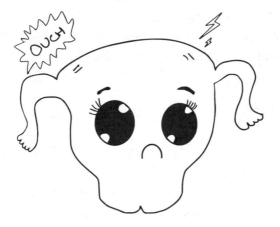

Every single month, your brain instructs your body to develop eggs, in the hope that one of these will be fertilized by a sperm. If that egg is fertilized, it goes to the uterus and becomes a pregnancy. If that egg is not fertilized, the uterus sheds off its inside lining in a period. And then the cycle starts over again. To let out all the endometrium that has been built up, the uterus has to squeeze itself like a lemon. We have some special chemical substances released by the body, called prostaglandins, that help the uterus squeeze itself. This causes the cramps we have when we are on our period. Taking a painkiller can help reduce the effect of these prostaglandins, and reduce the pain you might experience. It's totally chill to take a painkiller, and don't let someone tell you some bullshit about how taking a painkiller makes you weak. If you are in pain, take that painkiller; it will not make you infertile in the future, it will not make your uterus dry, and it will not cause cancer. With that said, if your pain is not relieved by painkillers, you should see a doctor. There can be several underlying conditions, like endometriosis, which can cause incredibly painful periods. There are treatments available for such conditions, so why suffer in silence?

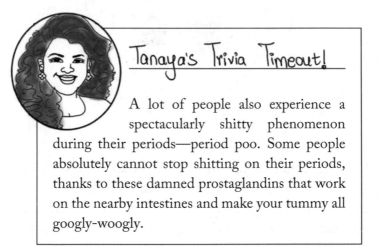

Tanaya's Trivia Timeout!

A lot of people also experience a spectacularly shitty phenomenon during their periods—period poo. Some people absolutely cannot stop shitting on their periods, thanks to these damned prostaglandins that work on the nearby intestines and make your tummy all googly-woogly.

You might also notice brown blood towards the start or end of your periods; this is nothing to worry about, and happens because the acidity of the vagina digests (oxidizes) the blood that your body is releasing. When you're having a normal flow, there is a fair amount of blood that the vaginal pH can't really affect much. But towards the start or end of your period, when you have a smaller amount of blood exiting the uterus, the acidity of the vagina can oxidize it, the same way iron oxidizes to rust, and make your period blood brown. It's just a natural variation in your cycle, not something to freak out about. Bright red, dark red, and brown period blood are pretty usual. What's unusual is when people start saying that pink period blood indicates estrogen dominance and other such things. That is actually bullshit dominance—you cannot predict your hormonal status from the colour of your period blood. Don't get overwhelmed trying to find fifty shades of red on your pad; we have no scientific evidence to say this pink-blood orange-blood stuff means anything.

Aside from the colour variations, you could also find clots in your period blood. Many people experience this—remember, the entire inside lining of your uterus is shed during the period. It's like peeling your skin off, but on the inside. So sometimes, there can be mucus, skin cells, and blood that can come out in clots. Usually, our vagina secretes a substance called fibrinolysin that helps keep our period blood liquid. But if you are having a heavy period, this small amount of fibrinolysin can fall short, and the blood can start clotting. Think of it like this: If you are making soup from those packaged soup powders you get in the market, you need to add water to make it soupy and delicious. Say you have 200 g of soup powder and you need to add 1000 ml of water to make a big bowl of soup. This will work great if you have 1000 ml of water, which will keep your soup runny and soupy. But, if you now suddenly have 500 g of soup powder, but only have 1000 ml of water, your soup will be thick and lumpy. The same way, we have enough fibrinolysin in our bodies to keep the blood from clotting. But if there is a heavy period, this fibrinolysin may not be enough, and some of the blood can clot. If you consistently experience big clots and heavy bleeding, you can speak to your doctor to figure out some options to reduce your flow.

Speaking of soup, contrary to what a lot of people suggest, there is no harm in eating sour or spicy food while on your periods. If you like spicy achaar, have it. If you like khichadi, have it. Oh, and please feel free to wash your hair whenever you like. I have heard from some patients that they are told to either not wash their hair on their period at all, or only wash it on the third day, or only wash it under the light of a full moon streaming through a banana tree (just kidding). There is no logic or science behind this; have a shower whenever you like and wash as much of your body as you like. Periods can be a ridiculously annoying time as it is, no need to add extra unnecessary rules on top.

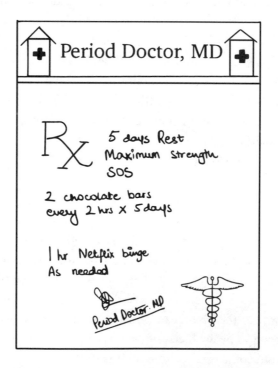

Period Doctor, MD

Rx 5 days Rest
     Maximum strength
     SOS

2 chocolate bars
every 2 hrs x 5days

1 hr Netflix binge
As needed

Period Doctor. MD

In fact, some of the more 'sinful' pleasures can be really helpful for your period pain. Dark chocolate has been shown to actually help you battle period pain. I'm talking about at least 70 per cent dark chocolate, not sugary milk chocolate. Although you can do that too if it makes you happy—periods suck and chocolate is delicious. Who am I to stop you? Dark chocolate contains a lot of magnesium, a mineral that works on muscles to help relieve cramps. (This is also why *kala namak* is used for muscle cramps, as it contains a lot of magnesium). You can throw in an orgasm on top to make your dark chocolate experience better. Seriously, orgasms can help you relieve period pain. We have a lot of research to back this claim up. Orgasms help you relieve stress and release feel-good hormones like serotonin and dopamine, which make you feel good and help relieve the pain. Additionally, an orgasm draws a lot of blood into your pelvis, which can help ease your cramps. Just whip out your vibrator, (or your fingers, or whatever you like) and go for the good vibes. In fact, you can even have sex on your period! Just make sure you spread down a towel to avoid your bedroom looking like a crime scene, and you're good to go.

Eat whatever you like, take painkillers, give your body rest, and just chill. Periods can be annoying and painful, but they're not toxic nuclear waste. I'm not exaggerating when I say that. We've treated menstruating people very badly throughout history. For example, in Nepal, they used to follow the traditional practice of *chaupaadi*, where menstruators would be sent off to live in a separate hut during their periods. This would make them feel ashamed about their body, and put them at risk of things like freezing to death (yep, that happened) or being bitten by venomous scorpions (that also happened), because of a completely natural and not at all dangerous phenomenon. Imagine being separated from your family and sent away to live in a small hut every time you had a runny nose—it makes no sense! Thankfully, in 2005, the practice was banned. But we still have to work hard towards unlearning all the shame that has been ingrained into us regarding our periods.

Period blood is not dangerous. It's not toxic. We believed these things when we didn't know enough about science and the human body. But scientists have actually conducted research to prove that period blood is not toxic. It's the exact same blood that flows through our veins. While most cultures have a shame-y relationship with periods, some cultures do have a really period-positive outlook. For example, did you know that in Japan, when you have your period for the first time, they throw you a big party? Everyone joins in and the family and guests eat red beans and rice, celebrating you and your period. Or how there is a whole festival called Ambubachi Mela that happens at Kamakhya Devi temple in Assam, where they celebrate the Goddess's period. Or how in certain parts of south India, we have the *ritushuddhi* or half-sari ceremony (known by many different names across India), where you're gifted a new sari and all of your friends and family come together to celebrate and have a bloody awesome party. If all that wasn't wholesome enough for you, let me come in with this: the sexual love of periods is called menophilia and there is a subcategory of porn called 'red rhapsody' for people who are really into period sex.

Or if all of this doesn't cheer you up, you can always think of these lyrics: 'Remember when NASA sent a woman to space for only six days and they gave her . . . 100 tampons. And they asked, "will that be enough" cuz they didn't know if that was enough.'

(P.S. That's an actual brilliant song by Marcia Belsky that you can listen to on YouTube. When the first American woman, Sally Ride, was sent to space for six days, the literal rocket scientists at NASA sent her with 100 tampons, not knowing if that was enough.)

13

Period Products

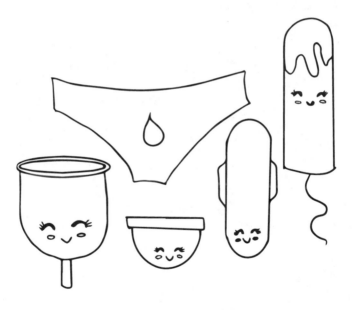

It's weird to be talking about this because until a few years ago, we didn't really have options in terms of period products. It was either pads, or errr . . . pads. No, wait, it could also be nothing. And a large percentage of our country continues to use absolutely nothing (or rags/leaves/ash—yes, ash!) for managing their periods. But in terms of actual products, we've mostly had only pads.

Until a few years back, that is.

Now we have a veritable avalanche of ways to manage periods—plastic pads, organic cotton pads, reusable pads, panty liners, tampons, Cannabidiol (CBD)-infused tampons, menstrual cups, menstrual discs, period panties—everything under the sun! Now, this can obviously be quite intimidating for someone who has periods. It's the opposite of a kid in a candy shop situation. How do you choose the right product? How do you choose what variety of the right product works best for you? Are they safe? Are they doctor recommended? Will they make you infertile? Will they give you infections? There are a lot of questions and a lot of answers, so let's break it down bit by bit. *Matlab, kaafi* overwhelming. If you need a refresher on your periods, please refer to the previous chapter to refresh your memory because I AM GOING TO QUIZ YOU. No, seriously, let's have a quiz.

1. Why do periods happen?
   A) If you don't get pregnant, the uterus sheds the endometrium two weeks after ovulation (aka your uterus is angry that you did not give it a baby)
   B) Because Mother Nature hates us
   C) Periods help let out toxic blood from the body every month
2. Are periods meant to be painful?
   A) Yeah, it's normal to be in absolutely debilitating pain
   B) Yeah, cramping is normal but if it is extremely painful, you should see a doctor

    C) No, period cramps are a sign that something is wrong
        with your uterus

3. Does missing a period always mean pregnancy?

    A) Oh yeah, it's baby time!

    B) No way, it's not a pregnancy

    C) It could be a pregnancy, or hundreds of different
        things like stress, hormonal imbalance, or just a
        late period

Okay, so the answers are 1A (and B), 2B, 3C.

Now that you have been a good kid, gone back and read the period chapter, and scored 100 per cent on this quiz, let's go ahead and talk about different period products.

Pads

Pads or sanitary napkins are the most commonly used period product across the world. They are kinda like diapers for your period—you take the pad, stick it on your panties, and let it absorb all the blood that leaks out. Some pads also come with wings, not to fly, but to help secure your pad snugly onto your panties. They contain a light glue on the back that helps them stay put on your underwear, even if you don't, (I mean, your pad doesn't) have wings. Pads are safe, if used properly, affordable, and easy to access. I frikkin' love pads! There is a 99.99 per cent likelihood that you will be able to find them at your local *kiraane ki dukaan*, and that the shopkeeper will wrap the packet of pads in two layers of newspaper, and then a plastic bag, before handing it over to you.

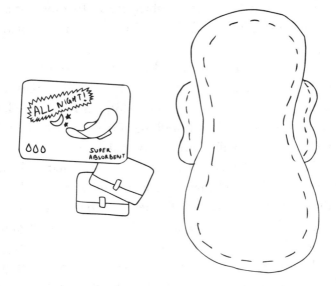

Pads are made up of three basic layers: the bottom-most plastic sheet; an inner core made of some synthetic material (with or without an absorbent gel), and a top perforated layer. The bottom layer is made of plastic and keeps the blood contained inside the pad. They would become kinda useless if the blood leaked out onto your panties, no? The reverse side of this layer has the glue and wings. The core layer is usually made of cellulose, and sometimes has a special gel core that is better at absorbing blood. The top layer has a kind of a *jaali* situation happening—there are small holes that allow the blood to reach the absorbent core, while separating your skin from the absorbent core and keeping you dry. (For some reason the song *Choli ke peeche kya hai* is playing in my mind as I describe this). We've had many, many revolutions and upgrades in Pad Technology, which means that the materials used in your pads are safe for use, and it's perfectly okay to use pads.

You might have seen hundreds of internet articles that say that pads cause cancer, that they contain toxins, and that they are terrible for you. Scary shit, eh? It's hard to have this conversation without talking about dioxins. Popular internet articles will confidently tell you that pads are awful because of their dioxin content. But what is dioxin? Dioxin is a chemical that does many, many things, but its claim to fame is that it is formed as a by-product of the process of bleaching the cotton and rayon fibres that go into your pads. It's a chemical that is a recognized carcinogen, which means it has established cancer-causing properties that affect humans and animals. So, of course, it's only reasonable that people are concerned about carcinogens in the bleached cotton used in pads. What the popular internet articles forget to mention is that the amount of dioxin released from sanitary pads is so minimal that it doesn't hurt you. In fact, you are at a significantly higher risk of absorbing more dioxin from the environment and your food, since it's widely present everywhere. (Thank you, pollution!) Pads are a reasonable choice for a lot of people, so if they work for you, don't fall for the internet rumours about cancer. Pads are nice and inexpensive, and pretty damn good at managing periods. What you might find interesting is how a lot of these pads-are-bad articles are written by companies that make period products (other than pads, d-uh) and also subtly end with a link to buy some product from them. Shady, no? It's a classic scaremongering technique to get you to drop your beloved pads, which you have been using for years without problems, and switch to their more expensive product. Marketing is evil.

That's not to say pads are perfect; they come with their own problems. A lot of people in the hot and humid environment of our country (and especially the hot and humid environment of our nether regions, hehe) develop nasty fungal infections when using pads. The top perforated layer can also cause painful chafing on the thighs and vulva, as it constantly rubs against the soft intimate skin. Like me, a lot of you would have memories of waddling like a penguin while wearing a pad, on your period, thanks to painful and irritated inner thighs. If the awkward penguin walk wasn't bad enough, you must also be careful to change your pad within eight hours (soaked or not) to prevent the growth of harmful bacteria and to keep yourself safe. Some people find the smell of pads unpleasant, which can be annoying. Although I'm gonna be your annoying science friend and point out that that smell develops from blood being exposed to air and getting digested (oxidized), not from the pad itself. Some pad manufacturers add fragrance to their products to cover this smell, although doctors strongly advise against using scented feminine hygiene products (what a weird term, by the way) as they can cause irritation, allergies, or worst of all, disrupt the delicate pH balance of the vagina. *Lo, aur* infection. On top of *all* this, there is the issue of disposal. The plastic problem that comes from disposable pads is too depressing for me to talk about, so I will conveniently skip it. (hey, I'm a human doctor, not a plastic doctor) . . . but thankfully, there are alternatives.

Reusable cotton pads are a popular choice. They're the same kind as regular pads, except they're made of cotton cloth so you can wash and reuse your pad, and no waste is generated (except when you decide that the cotton pad is too worn out to be used any longer, of course). This helps address the plastic waste problem, and also doesn't involve inserting anything into the vagina. A lot of people use and enjoy using their cotton pads, and why should they not? They're safe to use, cheap (other than the one time investment), don't come with pad rashes, and can even be made at home. Imagine upcycling your favourite dress into a new pad! If you are going to use them, make sure you clean your pad properly after use and dry it in the sun to help kill the germs. (yes, the sun is really kickass!).

There is a huge reason for pads being so beloved—they don't have to go *inside* your body in any way. They are perfect for people who feel anxious about inserting anything, and for people who are worried about damaging their hymen (more on that later). If you are okay with inserting something into the vagina, tampons and menstrual cups are two great options. Personally, I am a huge menstrual cup fan, so I will probably be talking about that for the next 15 paragraphs (okay, I promise I won't actually do that), so let's start with tampons.

Tampons

Tampons are small, disposable, cylinder-shaped thingies, made of rayon or cotton (or both) that absorb menstrual blood. Think of it like a cotton plug that you would insert into your nose if your nose were bleeding, except you put this inside your vagina. (My elderly millennial audience might remember a really funny scene from *She's the Man*. The vagina holds it in place for you securely, while all the blood flowing out of your uterus is absorbed nicely. There is a small string hanging at the end that you can use to pull the tampon out when it's soaked, or when it's time to change your tampon.

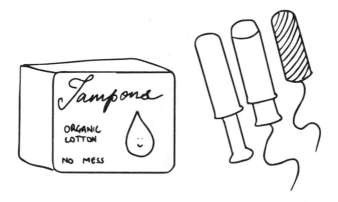

They do a really good job of absorbing menstrual blood and are a pretty cool option if you want to go swimming on your period, or just don't like pads. Some tampons come with a cardboard or plastic applicator, which can be helpful in insertion, but they're not necessary (*abhi plastic ki burai kari and now you want to get more plastic*?). They come in a large variety of absorbing capability, all the way from light, to medium, to super, to ultra- mega-super something (not the actual terminology). And this is where the problem with tampons can come in. The super-mega-ultra tampons, or even super tampons, are linked with a deadly infection called toxic shock syndrome (TSS).

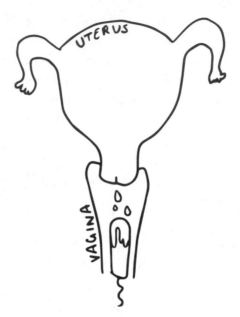

Essentially, because they're so good at soaking up blood (they're not called super absorbent for nothing), they also end up absorbing the natural vaginal discharge, which is essential to maintain a healthy vagina. This causes dryness and a change in the environment and pH of the vagina, which can be really bad for all the good bacteria that live inside your vagina and keep it healthy. This can instead encourage some infection-causing bacteria to grow. Additionally, sometimes when taking a tampon out, there can be tiny micro cuts in the walls of the vagina, since all the nice and natural lubrication is gone. While we don't fully understand exactly how tampons cause TSS, these two things are considered important reasons. Although rare, TSS is a medical emergency that presents with a fever, diarrhoea, and a sudden rash across the body. BE AWARE of this if you are using super-absorbent tampons. Or better yet, just get the low-absorbency tampons, wash your hands every time, and remember to change it within six to eight hours, even if it's not fully soaked. *Kaafi simple hai, matlab.* I'd also recommend sticking to some other period product when your flow is light, so you avoid causing that vaginal dryness. Wait, here's the strangest part—tampon use is not the only thing that can cause TSS, it can even happen from something like an infected wound. Yeah, it's wild. Basically, the whole world is really scary and messed up, so YOLO it. If tampons float your boat, use them, but use them safely.

Phew, that was some scary sounding stuff. The idea is obviously not to scare you, but to help you better understand your body and stay safe. Which brings me to my next option, which is so shrouded in mystery and misunderstanding that many people run away from it (even though it's a seriously kickass option). Let's talk about menstrual cups. (Wooohoooo!)

Menstrual Cups

A menstrual cup is a device made of medical grade silicone (this is a soft, flexible material that doesn't react with our bodies) that sits inside the vagina, and collects (instead of absorbing, like pads and tampons) period blood. The rim of the cup has several tiny holes in it which make a vacuum seal and hold the cup in place. They're the only menstrual product that can be worn for longer than eight hours (up to twelve hours, so you can conveniently get drunk, and not wake up panicking in the middle of the night about changing your pad or tampon) and last long (really long, ting tong). Most cups last at least five years, and some even for up to ten years. At the end of their lifetime, you can just burn your cup, or return it to the manufacturer for recycling. It's seriously low waste.

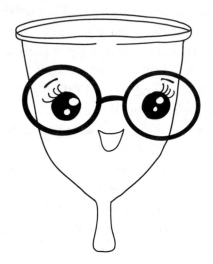

While buying a cup can feel like a really expensive investment to begin with, they turn out to be cheaper than other period products in the long run. A decent cup costs anywhere between Rs 500 to Rs 4,000, which although feels ridiculous initially when you compare it with the cost of a Rs 8 pad (with wings), it turns out to be cheaper in the long run. I actually did the math to break this down. So, we need to change our pad within 8 hours, which means 24/8 = 3, i.e, you'll use a minimum of 3 pads per day. Now 3 pads per day for 4 days is 12, and so, we'll use an average of 12–15 pads per period.

So, a standard pack of 50 pads (50/15 = 3.333) will last you around 3 cycles, which means you'll need 4 packs per year. One packet of 50 pads costs around Rs 360, which over a year (of 4 packs) comes to Rs 1440. An average menstrual cup is a third of that price! Phew, that was a lot of math!

So, yeah, I am really keen on driving home the fact that cups are actually cost-effective. The menstrual cup market has really boomed over the past few years, so there is a huge variety of sizes, shapes, and colours that are available, which means that there is a cup for everyone! Seriously, anyone can use a cup. (yes, even *virgins*)! To insert, you can squat and take a deep breath in to relax (if you are tense, your muscles will be tense, and insertion will be hard), and gently insert the cup into your vagina. If you aren't flowing very freely, you might not be that wet, which can make the insertion a bit tricky. I recommend using some water-based lube. Please don't use oil or cold creams for this, since they can damage the cup. You can even use tap water to ease the insertion process. The first couple of cycles involve a bit of trial and error, but most people find the techniques that work for them within three to four months of using cups! If you are using the right size, you won't even realize you're wearing a cup, not even when you are going to the bathroom. Since the cup collects all the blood as soon as it exits your uterus, it doesn't quite come out of the vagina the same way. No more bloody toilets! If you do feel it, it's probably not inserted correctly. Taking it out and reinserting it should make all the difference!

Which brings us to the removal process, which is also very simple. Simply squat and relax, as you did for the insertion, and reach inside yourself to find the stem of the cup. DO NOT PULL THE STEM DIRECTLY. This can put a lot of pressure on your internal organs, which can be bad for them. Instead, use the stem as a rope, and climb your way up (Rapunzel style) until you find the base of the cup. Gently squeezing this base will release the vacuum (as air will blow out of the tiny air holes on the top rim of the cup) and you can gently pull your cup out, without hurting yourself. Obviously, there will be spills and there is going to be a small learning curve involved, but it's like learning how to ride a bicycle. You will get there eventually.

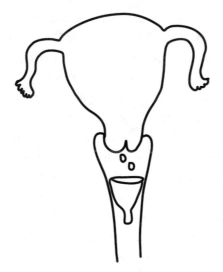

Now that its insertion and removal is out of the way, a menstrual cup is really pretty chill. A lot of people worry about losing the cup inside them—don't worry, your cup will not get lost inside you. Your vagina is not a black hole that will suck everything in; at the end of the vagina, there is the cervix. The cervix stops anything other than sperm from going into your uterus, and it's a thick, donut-shaped part, with a teeny tiny hole. You can't possibly push your menstrual cup past this. And that's it! That's the wonderful world of menstrual cups. I personally like doubling my protection by wearing a period panty along with my cup on heavy flow days to save myself from leaks and accidents.

Period Panties

But what are period panties now? Period panties are precisely what they sound like—they are just like regular panties that you can wear on your periods, which have an in-built pad to absorb all your period blood. It's a great option if you can't/don't want to insert anything vaginally but still want a sustainable period product. Like menstrual cups, these are also fairly expensive as an initial investment (ranging from Rs 1000 to Rs 3000 per underwear) but the cost works out eventually, as you can keep reusing them for a long time. You will probably need more than one panty—you obviously don't want to wear one pair throughout your period—which drives up the cost, but honestly, they are SO convenient! No sticking anything on your panties or inside yourself, the ease is seriously unreal. When you need to change them, just rinse your panties with cold water until the water runs clear, i.e., you can see no more blood and then hand wash or machine wash them like regular clothes. The ease makes it worth the money, truly. If nothing else, you can just buy one and use it as a backup with your tampon/cup on particularly heavy days—that's what I do!

We've come so far with the number of options we have for managing our period blood, and although we still have huge steps to take, I think we are now in a much better place menstrually, aren't we? So bloody good!

14

Masturbation

In the beginning, there was nothing.

Only Atum existed. Atum, the powerful Egyptian god of creation, existed all by himself. Simmering in his solitude, surrounded by nothingness, Atum decided to create the cosmos. And so, he masturbated. When he ejaculated, from his semen emerged the twins Shu and Tefnut. And the world was born. All the other gods were born of Shu and Tefnut, and the cosmos was created by the divine, magical act of masturbation.

According to ancient Egyptian mythology, the world was created by literally wanking it into existence. Every year, during a festival called the Feast of Nim, Egyptian pharaohs would honour this creation story. They believed that the ebb and flow of the river (and, therefore, the health of their harvest) was dependent on a good hand job. And so, in a very public ceremony, the pharaohs would disrobe and jack off into the river. Soon after, other men would follow, flooding the Nile with their cum. This is not an isolated river wank legend. In a similar story, the Sumerians believed God Enki created the great Tigris and Euphrates rivers by masturbating into their dry river beds. The rivers literally flowed from his semen, according to the legend. To the ancients, masturbation was an act that not just created whole ass rivers from cum, but it also enhanced virility and sexual power.

Masturbation is when someone touches their genitals with their hands (or other equipment) for sexual pleasure. It is a normal part of your natural sexual development. In fact, some research has shown that even babies masturbate inside the uterus (although some other research tends to disagree). Basically, we're quite enthusiastic about getting our rocks off. Human beings have been masturbating since the very dawn of time; we even have 30,000-year-old cave paintings to prove this. At some point in human history though, we decided that masturbation was a bad thing. For most of history, we haven't had such few and such healthy children; most babies would die earlier—in miscarriages, in childbirth, during infancy, and during childhood. In times of high infant mortality, when babies were dying left, right, and centre (yeah, history isn't quite as romantic as it may seem), wasting semen wasn't seen as a very intelligent decision. Semen was precious and important. We simply didn't know much about reproduction, since we still hadn't discovered the egg and the sperm, and that led to all kinds of bonkers ideas about boinking for babies. Some people believed there were tiny 'animalicules' living inside semen, some thought there were some strange vapours inside semen that made women pregnant, and some even assumed babies were made by men and transferred into women during sex!

Because of such ideas, people thought semen was sacred and special. In their mind, semen had magical life-giving properties! (But vaginal discharge is bad, y'know, the patriarchy tells us). So, for most of history between the ancient world and our modern world, masturbation was demonized. What was historically treated as a magical act at best and a slightly vulgar joke at worst, soon became taboo. 'Spilling the seed' was forbidden, and masturbation was thought to lead to all kinds of ailments, from causing hairy palms to blindness! It was only in the 1800s that the actual science behind baby-making was born (pun intended), and as you will see, all these concepts about the ills of masturbation are from before the 1800s. Science showed us the way, and debunked some of the bunk from before.

Some of the Victorian bunk said that epilepsy, tuberculosis, insanity, and a variety of other maladies were linked to masturbating your vital energy away. People started making a variety of contraptions and devices to stop themselves from getting turned on. Chastity belts, which were specially designed clothes with an actual physical lock on them, were worn by people to stop them from touching their genitals. Some inventively wore a spiked ring on their penis that would dig into the penis each time it became bigger in size, with an erection (the spikes were on the inside! Yikes!). In fact, our humble cornflakes were designed as an anti-masturbation food. A certain old-timey doctor believed that eating flavourful foods like meat and spices would make you super-duper turned on. Eating plain, bland food was the way to douse the horny hellfire inside your genitals, and so he came up with a dry, sugarless, flavourless food that decorates our breakfast tables to this day.

The doctor and his brother worked at a health resort where they started offering their newly minted cornflakes to the in-house patients. The cereal was a hit, but the brother wanted to add some good ol' sugar to the mix. The doctor disagreed; so the brother launched his own company to make the sugary breakfast cereal, and the most famous brand of cornflakes was born! In the meanwhile, the doctor continued to work prolifically as a doctor (a pretty good one at that) and continued his anti-masturbation crusade. The dude hated sex and masturbation so much that he even encouraged threading wires through the foreskin or rubbing carbolic acid on the clitoris to stop people from touching their sexy bits. He famously never consummated his marriage, spending his life writing about the dangers of masturbation, and adopted eight children.

Up until the late nineteenth century, anti-masturbation panic ran rife throughout the world. The twentieth century witnessed massive leaps in science, and our understanding of the human body. This led to a change in the way we view and understand sex, sexuality, and sexual health. We began to study and research sex, and found that, curiously, it was quite good for health! Masturbation is a very safe way to enjoy sexual pleasure, free from the risk of pregnancies and sexually transmitted infections, and completely in your hands (pun fully intended). It lets you learn about your own body, your likes and dislikes, and what turns you on.

There are SO many benefits to orgasms (through masturbation or sex), that I'm gonna have to make a (non-exhaustive) list of some of the coolest health benefits:

- Helps lower blood pressure
- Can help relieve stress (much better than a *sutta* break)

- Reduces the risk of prostate cancer (yepp, really)
- Makes your skin glow (the American cosmetic brand NARS has a best-selling blush called 'Orgasm' for good reason)
- Can help delay ejaculation for people with premature ejaculation
- Exercises your pelvic floor muscles, which makes them healthier and helps prevent erectile dysfunction
- Releases feel-good hormones such as endorphins, oxytocin, and dopamine, which also help you feel more connected with your partner
- Releases sleepy hormones like prolactin
- Releases hormones that also reduce your perception of pain
- Has been shown to relieve hiccups that absolutely won't stop
- May help relieve nasal congestion, according to a 2008 study

Basically, the consensus of the medical field is that masturbation is totally safe and harmless, and is good for your health.

Masturbation addiction is not a real diagnosis, no matter how much dudebros on the internet will tell you so. With that said, yes, there can absolutely be an abnormal relationship with masturbation where people do it compulsively. If it comes to a point where it interferes with your regular life, work, school; or it causes significant guilt or anxiety; or you're masturbating so much that you are chafing your genitals and irritating the skin, then it can be a problem. You could also be doing things described by the 1986 paper titled 'Masturbation Injury Resulting From Urethral Introduction of Spaghetti', which could be, um, dangerous. Doctors and mental health professionals can help overcome this compulsive behaviour. But masturbation does not lead to erectile dysfunction or premature ejaculation (in fact helps prevent it) and it does not drain you of your energy. Masturbation is healthy and normal.

There is a rare health condition called Post-Orgasmic Illness Syndrome (POIS) that some people can suffer from, where they become ill immediately after ejaculating. It sets in within minutes or hours of an orgasm, and can cause severe fatigue, muscle pain, headache, anxiety, itchy eyes, upset stomach, and various other symptoms. POIS can happen after masturbation, sex, or even after spontaneous night-time orgasms (night fall). It usually resolves within a week, but the symptoms return immediately if you ejaculate again within that time. We don't know too much about POIS at this point, but scientists are working hard on studying this condition. Since there are less than 100 cases recorded so far, it has been a bit difficult to study.

Human beings are not the only animals that masturbate. Animals are quite prolific in their jacking off, whether or not a partner is available. Bonobos are super horny, marmosets can suck their own dicks, orangutans have been seen to masturbate using twigs, spotted dolphins like to fuck sand, horses and elephants like to hit their dick against their abdomen for pleasure, and female chimps have been known to masturbate using mangoes, giving a whole new meaning to the sensuous *Aam Sutra* ad. The whole world is seriously amorously inclined.

But one thing we still don't really know is why we masturbate at all. Like what's the point, evolutionarily? Some evolutionary biologists think that masturbation helps us get rid of old sperm and clean the genital tract. When women masturbate, (which according to most studies, about 85 per cent women reportedly do) and have an orgasm, cervical fluid flows through the genital tract. This can help clear things up, and flush out the bad stuff. Since men are constantly making sperm all the time, if they don't ejaculate it, it gets reabsorbed by the body. However, if you just got rid of all that old sperm by masturbating, you'd have healthy, fresh sperm on top! This is just a theory though, and we don't really know why we evolved to jack off, other than the fun part.

Whatever the evolutionary purpose is, masturbation is fun, healthy, and super democratic—it's available to everyone, whether or not they have a partner. We have viewed masturbation for a long time as something done in shame, hidden away in a dark bedroom, in the dim light of a computer screen showing an X-rated scene. But maybe it's time to shed that crusty old persona of masturbation and embrace it for the lovely indulgence that it is.

Cum, let's walk into a sex-positive future.

15

Oral Sex

Use protection with oral sex.

Oh, and remember to have fun.

That's it. That's the chapter.

No, seriously. Go away now and read another chapter. Oral sex is fun, and can be a great way to enjoy yourself with your partner. Just remember to use condoms. Condoms are flavoured for this reason. Now go, have fun! You've already read everything you need to know about oral sex in other chapters, so I won't flog a dead horse.

16

Peaches

Oh, fruit blessed above all others
Good before, in the middle, and after the meal
But perfect behind!

—Francesco Berni

A peach is a soft, round, pinkish-orange fruit from the rose family. It has a thin, fuzzy skin, with a sweet-tasting flesh and a large stone inside it. The trees can be quite tall, almost 20-feet high, and have beautiful pale pink flowers in spring. Originally from China, peaches are now available and loved by people all across the globe. Justin Bieber has a whole song about them and how he gets them especially from Georgia. It makes sense since Georgia is often called the 'peach state' of the US. Throughout history though, the peach has often been a euphemism for another succulent fruit—a juicy, delicious, rotund, and plump fruit. I'm talking about the butt, and nothing but the butt. This speech about that peach was actually about the ass, and not at all a reach (I am a terrible poet).

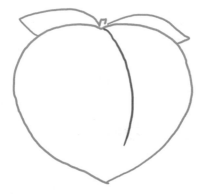

Beautiful behinds have fascinated humans across the centuries; you can find stunning posteriors in art, music, sculpture, pottery, and all forms of artistic expressions in the world. Heck, the Greeks even had a name for someone with a gorgeous ass—callipygian. Calli means beautiful (like calligraphy is beautiful writing) and pyga means butt. Try using that compliment on your next date, they'll love it. With our endless appreciation of butts, it's only natural that the next thing humans would do is to try to fuck it. And so, anal sex was born. And contrary to popular opinion, anal sex is not a modern invention. It has been practised for thousands of years, across many different civilizations and time periods. We have clay tablets from the 4000-year-old Babylonian civilization showing enthusiastic bum fucking; 2000-year-old pottery from the Peruvian Moche civilization showing passionate penetration in the behind (almost exclusively); intricate stone carvings in thousand-year-old Hindu temples depicting bum *waale mazze* happening between multiple people; and now, of course, the modern peach, brinjal, and water drops emojis, showing a deep and abiding love for bonk-bonk in the badadonkadonk that has survived throughout the existence of mankind.

Studies have shown that anywhere between 10 and 40 per cent people have reported tried anal at least once. And thanks to porn making anal sex more popular than ever, more and more people are willing to try it. But while anal sex can be really pleasurable if done right, it can also go catastrophically wrong. Like, it-can-kill-you wrong. So, it's important we learn about the butt, the different kinds of butt play, and how to do it safely without hurting ourselves or our partner(s). I'll also give you a Dr Cuterus checklist for safe anal sex at the end of this chapter, so make sure to keep it handy before you go in guns (or dicks) blazing.

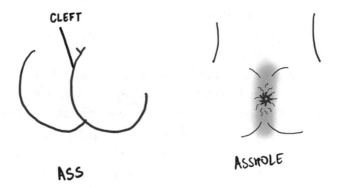

In case you don't know what anal sex is and the last three paragraphs have been confusing, let us clear that up. Anal sex is all kinds of sexual activities centred around the butthole— the place where your poop comes out from. If you look up the Wikipedia page on the 'anus' you will find it described as 'an external opening of the rectum located in the intergluteal cleft'. The rectum is a part of your intestine, so the anus is an opening at the end of your intestines. The intergluteal cleft is that line between two buttocks; like a hot and humid valley between the mountains of your butt cheeks. Inside this cleft, there lies a small, brown opening, called the anus. Anus in Latin means ring, and the anus is very much like a ring or a rubber band that stays closed to keep your poop inside. Think of it like a balloon—just as a balloon fills up with air, your rectum and anal canal are filled with poop. And at the end of the balloon, you have that ring-shaped thing that is tied up tightly to make sure air doesn't leak out, unless you loosen this ring-shaped thing. Your anus is the same! It acts like the end of the balloon to keep your poop inside and only lets it out when you relax the anus.

Actually, since we're talking about poop now, allow me to digress here: pooping is extremely interesting! We normally think that our body simply pushes poop out and that's how potty exits our body. Actually, what happens is that your body not just pushes poop out (by raising the pressure inside your abdomen and pushing), but the anus ring also lifts around that piece of poop. Instead of your anus opening up and the poop simply sliding out, what really happens is that the poop stays in the same place, but your anus is pulled up over it (and it's also pushed down by the raised pressure in the abdomen). Think of it like taking your socks off, your feet stay in the same place, but it's the sock that is moved down and allows your foot to be 'unsocked'. Poop works the same way: your anus is pulled up around a solid piece of potty, and then that potty, (which is now unsupported by the anus ring) falls into the toilet. Just as how you use your hands to pull off the socks, your anus uses a muscle called Levator Ani (which means the anus elevator, lol) and pulls it over the exiting poop.

Okay, back to the anus. So, while we use the anus mainly for pooping, there are a lot of sexual activities that dance around your butthole—you could kiss it and lick it (anal–oral sex), insert things inside it like fingers, toys, or the tongue or penetrate it with a penis. There can be a lot of fun that can be had playing with the butt, but there are some serious safety precautions that you must take to ensure a safe, pain-free, and enjoyable experience. You see, the anus is richly supplied with nerve endings; this means there can be more pain, and it can also mean more pleasure! The clitoris, penis, and anus have a shared nerve supply, and so a lot of people can have some really strong sexual stimulation from anal sex. Additionally, it can also indirectly stimulate the prostate for males, or the clitoris for females, and lead to orgasms for *some* people. The taboo nature of the act, coupled with the idea of complete domination and submission, can make anal sex mentally stimulating and erotic. And, of course, porn has made it super popular in the last few years too! No wonder lots of people want to try it!

So, where does one start? How does one dip a toe, so to speak, in the world of butt play? One of the most popular starter activities is anal–oral sex, or analingus. Here, one person makes out with their partner's butthole, and it can be pleasurable for both. Because you stimulate the rim of their asshole, it is also called rimming or a rim job. There is no penetration, the whole idea of pain is out of the window. Some people like to use this as an appetizer (lol, in more ways than one) to the main course of penetrative sex, but some people are just really into eating ass. Whichever way you like, if you are thinking about having anal–oral sex (hey, this is a judgement-free space, you do you), there are certain precautions to bear in mind. Because the butt is Poop Central, anal–oral sex can be a great way to not just accidentally touch poop with your mouth, but also catch infections. Everything from viral infections such as HPV, Hepatitis A, B, and C, to bacterial infections that cause diarrhoea to parasitic infections (worms) to sexually transmitted infections can all spread from anal–oral sex. The higher the number of partners you have, the higher the risk. In fact, one study has even shown an increased risk of throat cancer from unprotected oral sex, (of all kinds, genital or anal). So, always remember to wash your butt properly before anal sex to get rid of any leftover poopy bits, and making sure you use a dental dam between the anus and the mouth. This way, there is no direct contact between the mouth and the butt, so your risk of contracting an infection goes down dramatically.

If you'd like to graduate from the world of anal–oral sex, you can step up to penetrative anal sex. This is where you'd insert something into the anus: fingers, toys, or the penis. People tend to have very strong reactions to this sexual activity, so please feel free to skip this section if you'd like. If you're interested, please make sure you have a long and detailed conversation with your partner about this to make sure you are both enthusiastically on board before trying it out. While I recommend this for every sexual practice, this is doubly important with anal sex because there is an increased risk of injury and STIs. Unprotected anal sex is considered the *riskiest* sexual activity, so please be careful.

The reason why it's considered the riskiest is because of three main issues: lack of natural lubrication, the tightness of the anus, and the fragility of the tissue. Unlike the vagina, the anus does not make any natural lubricant to allow for penetration. This can cause unnecessary friction, pain, irritation, cuts, and injuries on penetration. Using an additional lubricant is *essential* for anal sex if you want to prevent these injuries. Lube is also helpful to make penetration easier, because the anal sphincter—the rubber band like muscle of the anus that helps keep your poop in— is quite tight, and inserting objects, especially the penis, can be painful and difficult. Lube adds some slipperiness to make this more comfortable, the same way lathering soap on your hands before you slide on a tight bangle helps. Forcing an object inside an unlubricated anus can be painful and can cause tears inside the anus. Not just that, since anal tissue is quite delicate, it's very important to treat it gently. Otherwise, it can have microscopic, (as well as large) cuts that increase the likelihood of sexually transmitted infections entering the bloodstream and infecting you. In fact, anal sex is associated with the highest risk of contracting HIV. And then, of course, there are the additional poo-poo related bugs that live in your butthole, so you can get infected cuts inside your butts (sorry, I had to!) if you go at it without lube. Just use lube, okay?

Just using lube is not enough though, you need to include condoms too. Not for preventing pregnancy, d-uh, but as protection from STIs. (It's really unlikely that you might become pregnant from anal sex). Avoid textured and ribbed condoms, as they can irritate the fragile inner lining of the anus. Instead, choose lubricated condoms, and apply extra lube on top—the wetter, the better! This is seriously helpful because the anus can be really tight and can cause the condom to slip off. Just use a condom, okay? If you get HPV (an STI) in the butt, it can cause anal cancer. Do you want cancer in your butthole? No? Then use a condom. Oh, and you must remember to change your condom if you change the hole: if you are going from anal to vaginal, or anal to oral, please change the condom. Going into the vagina directly from the anus can increase your partner's risk of getting a UTI (poo bacteria can cause pee infections), and going into the mouth directly from the anus, also called ass-to-mouth or A2M for short, can increase your partner's risk of throwing up (lol) and STIs. This advice is not restricted just to the penis, it also covers the use of toys. Cover your insertable sex toys with a condom, slather them in some slippy-slippy-lubey love, and change the condom if you share your toys with a partner. Share your love, your joys, your sorrows, but maybe not your STIs.

Just like a warm-up before lifting that 40-kg barbell is great to prevent injury, using a toy is a great warm up to get the bum-bum used to having things (other than shit) inside it. Work on gently easing the butthole muscles, get them to relax with smaller objects, and then insert your penis in there only after it's sufficiently warmed up. You're essentially training the butt muscles; booty building of a different kind. This is super important to prevent injury (and we all now know just how *chhuii muuii* the butthole is) and to make sure that the sexual experience is actually enjoyable, instead of, y'know, miserable and painful. Cuz sex is fun! Keep it fun! Do not hurt your partner (unless they're into it, in which case, slap the shit out of them!) by forcing stuff into the butt. Go slow, go easy. And if they're in pain, stop. Pain is a sign from the body that something is not right. Slow and steady wins the race, and all that shit, y'know.

Oh, and also, please don't just shove *anything* inside the butt—we have enough emergency room horror stories to last us a lifetime. Don't use sharp things (for the obvious risk of cuts in your butts), or glass objects (as they can shatter inside you, which . . . ouch!). Use toys that are easy to clean and have a flared base; this means use toys that have a thick bottom part so they are easy to withdraw. Because unlike the vagina, you can actually have stuff get lost inside the butt. The butt has this superpower of 'sucking' things up inside it, like a black hole. So, if you shove something long and smooth in there, say like a cucumber, it can get sucked inside and stuck. (I may or may not have seen a patient in the emergency room with this exact problem). If this cucumber had a wide part at the bottom, only the long upper part would go into the butt, leaving the thick bottom outside. You could easily grab this and pull the toy out. This is why butt plugs are shaped in that weird way, with a stand at the bottom. Not because they're wanting you to display it as a showpiece in your cabinet. (Although go do it if you want to! There is no shame in great sex!)

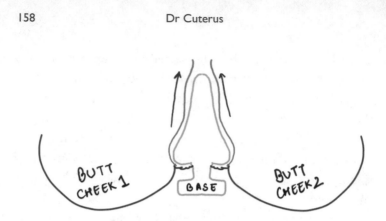

If you don't want to spend money on objects to shove in your literal asshole, fingers can be a great (and inexpensive) alternative. Remember to lube it up and keep your nails blunt and short (because again, cuts in your butts. Maybe I should rename the whole chapter this.). Just please don't get too inspired by porn and try to shove your whole hand in there. Because anal fisting is a thing. A thing I do not recommend. Anal fisting, when done by inexperienced individuals (or even experienced people for that matter) can cause such intense internal injuries that they can cause perforations in the intestinal walls and lead to death. In less severe cases, it can cause things like rectal prolapse, where the rectum falls out of the asshole, like an inside out sock (do NOT Google this, the images will keep you up at night) or faecal incontinence (poop leakage from the butt). Just don't put your fist in someone's rectum. Please.

Aside from all the things you should be using for safe anal sex, there are also some things you should not be using in addition to lightbulbs, and sharps, and all the fun stuff we've covered before. I'm talking specifically about the numbing creams you might find in the market that help make the asshole numb and anal sex pain-free. Please don't use them, because pain is your body's response to tell you that something is wrong. If peepee inside poopoo hurt, take out, no in. It means that the anus is not stretched out enough and requires more lube. Using a numbing cream there will numb your pain receptors, and you wouldn't know when things are going wrong. It's – the same way you have pain receptors on your hand that hurt when you accidentally grab the hot part of your hair straightener, so you drop it and prevent a burn. Pain is good (as the BDSM community will also tell you) and is meant to protect you. Don't try to numb the pain; instead use safe practices so it doesn't hurt in the first place.

Pain and all is okay, but what if it starts bleeding?! Blood is red, and red means danger, so bleeding means STOP. Bleeding is NOT normal, whether you're doing anal for the first or fiftieth time. If your ass is leaking blood from anal sex, that means something has gone wrong and you definitely have an injury. Do. Not. Continue. Penetration. Leave the bum-bum alone. And next time, follow my checklist to make sure this doesn't happen. And if you bleed from your bum-bum without the sex (it means you have haemorrhoids), it's probably best to leave the bum-bum alone anyway. Haemorrhoids are swollen blood vessels around the anus, and unless you are very experienced with anal sex, I wouldn't recommend knocking on that door.

Reading all that advice would have looked very different from what you might have seen in porn; after all, porn shows bare dicks being shoved into bleached assholes with no lube or warm up. Let this serve as your reminder that porn is entertainment, not education. Nobody has a dick that long, or lasts that long, and body parts don't look like that in real life. Oh, and people don't have hairless, light-coloured assholes. Porn star booties go through some rigorous beauty procedures to give them those red carpet-ready butts. Everyone has hair around their asshole, which is totally normal (Please don't try to shave your asshole. Not only will it involve folding yourself up in ambitiously pretzel-like yoga poses, but it can also cause, say it with me, cuts in your butts! And these cuts can get infected pretty badly, because poop). Waxing is also available for the butthole, but again, I do not recommend it. Butthole hair exists to prevent chafing between your butt cheeks, and protect your bum hole. Do you want a chafed, irritated asshole? Probably not. So, leave that hair alone, and remember to clean your ass in the shower, especially if you use toilet paper to clean up after you poop. Bits of toilet paper + sticky gooey poop can wrap around your ass hair and lead to the very interestingly disgusting phenomenon of dingleberries. It's called that because clumped up toilet paper with poop hanging on an ass hair looks like berries hanging on a tree. I urge you not to Google it, for your sanity. Wash your ass.

And while we're on that, you don't need to bleach your asshole either. Bleach is highly irritating, and if you have an inflamed, angry asshole, you will be walking around like an inflamed angry asshole. More so if you've shaved off your butt hair, and then put bleach on top. That's like irritation double *dhamaal*. It's normal for your butt and butthole to be darker than the rest of your body, don't worry about it. And don't bleach it. Your big, hairy, pigmented butt looks just the way Mother Nature intended.

The doctor's advice? Just keep it clean. Wash your ass in the shower. Eat a healthy diet high in fibre for your butt health and overall health. Always use protection, and don't get bothered about waxing and bleaching your asshole. It's the place where the sun don't shine, of course, it's gonna be dark in there. Too many people lose their sleep over the size of their ass; don't even worry about it. Big butts, small butts, all are good butts. You are a callipygian beauty.

P.S. Cuts in your butts.

Just wanted to put it in your head one last time.

17

Sexy Shopping

There is a HUGE market for sex products: toys, lubricants, performance enhancers, aphrodisiacs, cannabis-infused products . . . The list is endless! But what actually works? Is it all a gimmick? How do you decide between good products and bad products? Which products should you use together? What should you avoid? There is a cartful of stuff you can buy, so let me take you through them one by one. To make your sex journey smoother, let's start with lube (wink-wink, nudge-nudge).

Lubey Doobey Do

A lubricant is a liquid or gel that can be used to help reduce friction. Since sex is a very friction-y activity, lubes can make things nice and slippery. Think of yourself trying to wear a tight bangle on your wrist; you can keep tugging and pushing but it won't do much other than hurt a lot and give you rashes and burns on your hand. But throw on some soap or oil on that bad boy, and watch how quickly your bangle slides onto your wrist. Lubes do the same thing; they can help with penetrative sex, (vaginal or anal), they can also help with solo sex, and they can help with sex with toys. Lubes are like chocolate—they make everything better!

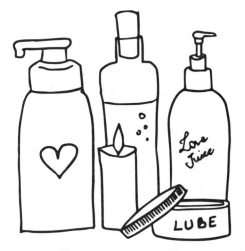

And just like you don't need a special occasion for chocolate, you don't need a special occasion for lube. You don't need to be dry to use lube. Lubes can be used even when you're producing enough natural lubrication. They can also be used during anal sex, since our butts don't make any natural butt lubricants. Lubes increase pleasure and sensitivity. Lubricant is not just for menopausal people, it's for everyone at all times.

There are three main types of lubes available in India: water based, silicone based, and oil based. They all have their own special advantages and disadvantages, so you can figure out what works best for your specific needs. With that said, avoid using saliva or Vaseline as a lube. Saliva dries quickly and may increase your chances of contracting STIs (if you don't use condoms) as well as increase your risk of getting a fungal infection. Vaseline contains oil, which is known to break down the latex of the condom. Additionally, it's not great for the vagina as it interferes with the vaginal environment and has been shown to double the risk of bacterial vaginosis. Leave the Vaseline for your lip balm only.

Water-based lubricants are made of . . . water. They're cheap, most easily available, and most dum-dum friendly. They can be used safely with toys and condoms, don't stain, are easy to wash off, and come in the widest variety. Silicone-based lubricants are great for people with allergies, since silicone is hypoallergenic. It's super slippery and lasts long, (so it's great for marathon sex sessions), and unlike water-based lubricants, can be used safely for shower sex! While you can use silicone-based lubes with condoms, they can destroy your silicone toys. Also, it needs soap and water to wash off, and can stain your sheets. Lastly, we have oil-based lubes. They last foreeeeever and can double up as massage oils. But they break down latex—so you can't use them with condoms—stain your sheets, need soap and water to be washed off, and increase your risk of fungal infections. If you are going to be using a natural cooking oil (like coconut oil), bear these things in mind. Also, use unrefined oil, and then don't use that jar for anything other than as sex oil. You don't want to cross-contaminate your food oil and your sex oil.

Now that we've established the main types of lubes, let's talk about the things you should avoid in your lube of choice. I don't recommend using flavoured lubes for oral or penetrative sex; instead, use it for playing with other parts of the body. Put some flavoured lube on your partner's tummy and lick it off. Put it on their knees and tickle them! Flavours, colours, and sugars can be irritating when used on the fragile genital skin. Some people can be highly sensitive to the 'sensations' inducing lubes—the warming, cooling, tingling kinds. If it has worked for you without any issues, sure, go ahead and use it. But if not, don't unnecessarily introduce those into your play routines. The basic rule of thumb is to avoid colours, flavours, sugar, and essential oils in your lube. Anything that goes into a cupcake should not go into your lube. Additionally, we have strong research to show that two compounds should be avoided: nonoxynol (a spermicide) and polyquaternium 15. They have been shown to increase your risk of HIV. I also don't recommend lubes that promise to make you last longer and contain numbing agents like benzocaine, because what the fuck is the point of sex if you're making your genitals numb?

Two of the most controversial ingredients in the lube industry (yeah, it's a multimillion dollar industry) are glycerine and glycerol. There is *massive* fear mongering in online educator circles about how these two sugary Gs are terrible and will give you fungal infections. The truth of the matter is we don't have enough evidence to say that yet. Some research shows that it increases your risk, while some research says that it has no effect. If you're prone to UTIs and fungal infections, it's best to avoid lubes that contain high amounts of glycerine and glycerol. What we do know is that you should avoid lubes that have a high osmolality; this means that they act like a sponge and can draw a lot of water out of tissue. This causes tissue dehydration, which makes your tissue fragile, and increases your risk of STIs. If it all sounds complicated, I'm sorry but I suck at chemistry, so I suck at explaining this. Basically, avoid 'hyperosmolar' lubes, i.e., that have an osmolality higher than 1200 mOsm/kG, and ones that have a high amount of glycerine or glycerol, until there is more research on this. If you're wondering how to find out the osmolality of lubes, a simple email to the manufacturer should help. Glycerine and glycerol do have a high osmolality, so avoiding these ingredients should be helpful.

Sexy Score - 5/5

So, lubes make sex better, and now you know how to use the right kind of lube. But how do you make sex better? Is there anything available that increases your sexual power? Across history, several aphrodisiacs have existed throughout the world that claim to make you better at sex and increase sexual desire. As per my penchant for destroying everything that sounds nice, allow me to destroy aphrodisiacs for you.

Aphrodisiacs

Aphrodisiacs are foods or ingredients that claim to stimulate sexual desire, increase lust, and fire up your passions. Stoke your fire for sexy times. Increase your hunger for boink-boink. Make you horny. Improve your skills at horniness. You get the drift. Aphrodisiacs are named after the Greek Goddess of love and sex, Aphrodite. Funnily enough, Aphrodite had a distinctly unsexy birth: her daddy, Uranus (I cannot write that without laughing) had his balls chopped off and thrown into the sea. From his chopped off balls mixing with the sea water, a beautiful goddess was born, Aphrodite. She grew up and became the literal goddess of sex, and so foods that make you want to do the sexy are called aphrodisiacs.

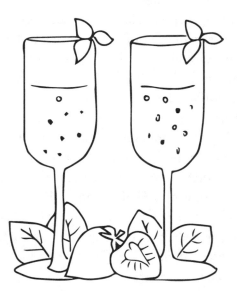

I mean, dude, we all know food is sexy. Food porn is a full-on thing. The licking and slurping of delicious food, some ketchup exploding over a juicy burger, the intoxicating smells of scrumptious chocolate, the hot sizzle on some *garma garam pakode*—all of this must be making your mouth water, na? Food has been sexy across the world throughout history. And some foods, like aphrodisiacs, have been thought to make you feel more passion. Generally speaking, there are certain categories of food that have been said to make you horny: rare and expensive items such as oysters, truffles, and saffron, foods that make you hot such as spices, ginger, and alcohol, food that looks like genitals such as avocado, pomegranate, and eggs, and actual genitals eaten as food, e.g., organs from animals.

This economic principle in food and sexy times is so strange—the sexual power of foods was controlled by supply and demand! Rare foods were thought to make you horny. And so, rare and expensive foods like champagne, caviar, oysters, and truffles have all been thought to make you better at sex. Hell, potatoes were once considered an aphrodisiac at a time when they were rare in Europe (although to be honest if my partner bought me fries, I would 100 per cent bang him). During the Middle Ages, oysters became a popular sex food and they even served pickled oysters in brothels! Casanova famously ate 50 oysters every morning for breakfast. In fact, his most famous seduction technique was to teach his object of desire how to eat an oyster. Oysters also look a bit like a vulva, so that helps, I guess?

We Indians also adore love drugs and potions. Everything from the *Kama Sutra* to the *Sushruta Samhita*, an ancient medical treatise on surgery, and the *Rig Veda* talk about kickass supplements that make you better at sex. The *Kama Sutra* even has a whole chapter on them, (surprising absolutely no one). Many Indian aphrodisiac recipes use some combination of milk, honey, ghee, saffron, and nuts. The whole *haldi doodh* on the *suhaag raat* suddenly makes a lot of sense, doesn't it? *Keeda jadi* and *shilajit* are well known for their 'power-enhancing' properties. Shatavari is another herb that is famed for boosting your libido. And then there are some very problematic aphrodisiacs like the ground-up horn of a rhino, the glands of a toad, or tiger penises.

But does the science stack up? Well, there is very little scientific evidence to say that any of these famed aphrodisiacs work. It seems to be a combination of placebo effect + no effect at all. If you're just eating some harmless oysters or having some milk, that's probably fine. But if you're buying a powder or pill that claims to make you sexually stronger, that can be a problem. Not only are they not proven to be helpful, but there are also some bigger risks—the supplement industry is not very regulated, so you could be consuming anything at all! It could be contaminated with prescription medications or toxic substances, which can cause dangerous side effects such as liver toxicity, hallucinations, insomnia, and kidney damage. Even worse, some of the animal-derived aphrodisiacs can create a market for animal poaching, especially for endangered animals such as the rhinoceros. Illegal wildlife trading and the ruthless killing of animals is not worth an extra two minutes of sex.

Sexy Score - 0/5

(Eat your fruits and veggies though, they're good for you!)

Lingerie

When I was in medical school, I had a dear friend whose roommate used to steal her lingerie. No, I'm not making this up. She really did. Being the awful friend that I am, I made a song to tease my friend about this. She was not happy, but she did laugh a lot. The lyrics went like this:

Ishq Mohabbat (ting ding ding)
Pyaar ki baatein (ting ding ding)
Bekaar ki baatein (ting ding ding)
Hum toh chaddi shehezaade!
Hey! Lady!
Le le meri chaddi ko,
Hey! Lady!
Bra ki sochenge kal ko

I am extremely proud of this beautiful parody and still sing it to my friend to this day. If you're also a *chaddhi shehezaada* and want to learn more about lingerie, allow me. There is a surprisingly wide variety of underwear available in the market. The rules are very simple: wear comfortable undies that fit you well, avoid wearing super tight underwear, and change your underwear regularly. No, I don't mean that you need to buy new *chaddis* every few months. I mean put on fresh ones every day. Cotton panties are great, especially in the hot and humid Indian weather. Synthetic materials are probably okay, but we don't have a lot of scientific evidence on how good or bad they are. Theoretically, synthetic fabrics will trap more moisture and heat, so I personally recommend that you limit your usage of synthetic fabrics. We have enough heat and moisture down there anyway thanks to Indian weather. If you have a vagina and are wearing synthetic panties, look for ones that have a cotton lining on the crotch, i.e., the part that touches your vulva lips. If vaginal discharge bothers you, you can use panty liners.

Best undie competition

If you own a penis, keep your balls cool by wearing boxers. Briefs are fine, but boxers are better for your nuts. If you own a vagina, the cut of the panty doesn't matter since you're not concerned about fried-egg testicles inside your underwear. Thongs are fine; they are not known to increase your risk of vaginal infections. Whatever genitals you have and whatever kind of undies you wear, going undie-free at night can make you feel nice and aired out. I recommend skipping the undies and wearing loose cotton pyjamas at night.

Sexy score - 5/5

This underwear advice is quite plain, simple, and unsexy. Thankfully, the undie world was changed forever in 1975 when two entrepreneurs from Chicago created 'candypants', the world's first edible underwear! It seriously took off, earning hundreds of thousands of dollars! People wanted delicious panties, and they wanted them bad. In fact, while researching this book, I happened to talk to a very lovely person from a condom brand who mentioned to me that India was one of the largest consumers of edible panties in the world. The *rosogolla*-loving state of West Bengal leads the charts, with Odisha following closely behind. I haven't found any evidence to back this up yet, so we will take this with a pinch of *sondesh*. Since we apparently love to pump our hard-earned rupees into edible panties, I do recommend being careful with them. Since they are literally made of sugar, they can increase your risk of fungal infections, throw off your vaginal pH, and increase your risk of bacterial vaginosis. Not to mention that they must be super sticky and a mess to clean up. It's great for a one-time novelty thing, I guess. But don't use edible panties on the regular. Just buy some candy—we have a better variety there. You could try edible bras though.

Sexy score - 1/ 5 (one point for novelty)

We have all learnt to begrudgingly wear bras, whether we like it or not. Thankfully, there has been a small revolution and a lot of people are choosing to go bra-free now. If you want to learn more about bras, you can go to the chapter on breasts that explains whether or not you need a bra. I'm here to give you the low-down on bras.

Sexy Score - This is a matter of personal choice; so I won't score this.

Toys

If you think sex toys are some new-fangled contraption, let me tell you that the oldest sex toy discovered is 28,000 years old from a cave called Hohle Fels in Germany. This is literally from the Stone Age—the old Stone Age precisely. This is so frikkin old that back then even agriculture hadn't been established yet; we were still hunter-gatherers. Human beings have been such proper horn dogs that we made sex toys even before we learnt how to grow food!

Sex toys are, well, toys that can be used with sex. They can make sex more pleasurable, help with solo pleasure, help with couple pleasure, and even be therapeutically used as medical devices. There are many different kinds of sex toys such as vibrating toys (which can be used on any body part, but are usually used on genitals), dildos (meant for penetration), anal toys (meant specifically for anal sex), penis toys, (such as cock rings that are worn around a penis and can even vibrate), and masturbation sleeves (in which you can insert a penis). A wide variety of toys is available, and describing them would make up a whole book, so I will leave you to do your own research.

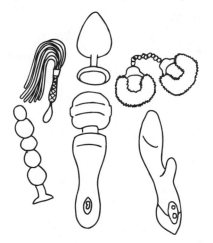

Whatever kind of sex toy you like, there are some basic safety precautions to follow. Remember to wash them with soap and water every time before using. If you're sharing penetrative toys, cover them with condoms, and remember to use lube, especially for anal sex. I recommend buying toys made from body-safe and non-porous materials such as plastic, metal, or 100 per cent silicone. Porous toys have small holes in them (like the pores on your face) where bacteria can live and cause infections. Using smooth, non-porous materials cuts down your risk of infections. Items made of polyvinyl chloride (PVC), jelly rubber, and silicone blends tend to be porous. It's for this reason that you shouldn't use household items as sex toys. Plus, they can cause injuries.

My favourite historical sex toy? An incredible and simultaneously terrifying 1000+ year-old Chinese sex toy—a cock ring, made by sewing goat eyelids into a circle, (with the eyelash hair still on there for some furry pleasure).

Sorry, not sorry.

Sexy score - 5/5 (not the goat-eyelid toy, obviously)

Foetus Deletus

18

The History of Birth Control

Now, let's step into Imagination Land for a second. Picture this: you're a beautiful young girl with big dreams, a hot husband, and a lovely house. It's a sunny, breezy afternoon, and you're thinking of a bottle of wine, some sexy music, and some alone time with your hubster tonight. Oh, by the way, this little imagination exercise is set 3500 years ago, in Ancient Egypt. So, yeah, you're walking along the Nile in your beautiful, flowy Egyptian cotton dress, sexting your man (in hieroglyphs?) on your ancient Egyptian cell phone, telling him you're feeling really horny and want to do bonk-bonk with him tonight, behind the pyramids. He's excited, you're excited, and so you head home to prepare. You have a long bath, wash and style your hair, put flowers in it, shave your legs, and stuff your vagina with crocodile dung. Wait, what?! Yes, croc poop. One of the most popular Ancient Egyptian contraceptives used to be a mix of plant slime (ew) crocodile dung (double ew but also wow) that would be stuffed into your vagina and help prevent a pregnancy. Only the Ancient Egyptian gods knew how!

Thankfully, since then, contraceptive methods have had a proper glow-up. From the early days of stuffing the vagina with various concoctions and swallowing weird herb mixes, to the now (incredibly) more palatable version of popping a pill, we have come a long way. Humans have forever wanted to do the sexy times without the risk of accidentally making babies with it. And so, in our endeavour for baby-free sexy times, we've come up with some seriously interesting solutions. Let's take a walk through history and learn the story of contraception. It's a very interesting tale; inextricably and surprisingly linked to women's harassment and also empowerment through the centuries.

Our story begins 4000 years ago in Ancient Mesopotamia and Ancient Egypt, where they used a paste made of acacia fruit mixed with honey and dates, which sounds delicious, as contraception. A piece of cotton would be covered in this paste and shoved inside the vagina, like an ancient tampon. And they also had the famed crocodile dung mix, of course. We Indians got in on that party too, but in true grand old Indian fashion, we used elephant dung instead of crocodile dung. We're nothing if not majestic, after all. Around 2000 years ago, the Greek gynaecologists Soranus (which absolutely does not sound like sore anus, no siree) suggested that blocking the cervix with a mix of resin, honey, olive oil, and lead, and then sneezing *super* hard after sex would help you not get pregnant. This sounds very . . . interesting, but what if you could not sneeze on command?

And then we have the star of the ancient contraceptive world. Say hello to Silphium, the ancient plant considered so important that it was worth its weight in silver! It was loved by the Egyptians, Greeks, Romans, and Minoans, who for six centuries, reportedly consumed Silphium seeds in a juice, which apparently worked as a natural contraceptive, every month. Silphium would be traded like a precious commodity; in fact, it was so valuable that the Cyrenians put an image of Silphium seeds on their currency. It was also considered an aphrodisiac—if you Google Silphium, you will notice that its seed looks curiously heart-shaped. This may not be a coincidence because some scholars think that's where the modern image of a heart symbol comes from! Isn't that incredible? Silphium allowed people to make love in a carefree fashion, and to this day, we (maybe) use it as a symbol of love. How utterly adorable! But as anyone who has been in a suffocating relationship will know, too much love can also be a bad thing. These guys loved Silphium so much, they basically consumed it into extinction.

While we don't quite know too much about Silphium (now that it's extinct), the one thing we do know is this: Silphium happens to be a relative of asafoetida, which is better known as *heeng* in India. Maybe *heeng* has some baby-controlling properties? And that's how it became so popular in our cuisine? Who knows! We have used other plants for birth control though, the most popular among them being Queen Anne's lace, aka *jangli gaajar* (wild carrot). Apparently even good ol' Hippocrates was a fan of this, and wrote about it more than 2000 years ago. There are some jokes to be made about how carrots are phallic and how it's ironic that they're linked with contraception but I will skip it cuz it's just too easy. We're talking cool history shit right now! Talking of cool Indian history, it turns out we've been using a variety of contraceptives, usually some herbal mix, through the years! They are listed in some of the texts of Vatsyayana (the fab dude who wrote the *Kama Sutra*) and other *desi* sex manuals like *Ananga Ranga*, and *Rati Rahasya* (literally meaning Rati's Mysteries, Rati being the Hindu goddess of sexual pleasure).

In contrast, the West was definitely not a fan of this contraception nonsense. And once again, for this we must thank our most famous anti-birth-control sponsor, the Church, which deemed it 'immoral' to try to prevent a pregnancy. In 1484, Pope Innocent VIII issued an official document that said witches were real and we should kill 'em all. Women who killed infants inside the womb, i.e., performed abortions, or hindered conceiving, i.e., used contraception, were bad bitches, sorry, witches, and would be hunted and burnt. And so, using contraception became deadly in more ways than one.

But it's not like that stopped us. For the next 500 years, more methods and tips and tricks were tried, but more secretly. *Matlab bhai try toh humne sab kuch kiya hai*—even lemons and Lyzol. Lemons are an incredibly popular *gharelu nuskha* for everything under the sun, so it's no surprise that lemons were also used as contraception. Most famously, Casanova—the most legendary fuckboi of all time—used half a squeezed lemon like a little cap to cover his partner's cervix. To which I say: (*a*) ouch! and (*b*) the man must have been really smart because lemon juice would surely kill *some* of the sperm and also change the vaginal pH. (Do not try this at home please. No lemons in vaginas. Just no.)

Until the 1820s, we only knew about the sperm: sperm gave life, and the uterus was just the house. It was only in 1827 that the female egg was discovered and the female contribution to baby-making was recognized. With reproductive knowledge that rudimentary, it was no surprise that at this time an average woman in the US would get pregnant about fifteen times, and have at least eight live children. While early birth control was often toxic and dangerous, it was still better than getting pregnant, considering death during childbirth was so incredibly common. Thankfully, things were about to get better. And then worse. And then better again. But still bad.

The 1920s brought on a gender revolution like no other: women wanted to vote, they wanted to work, and they wanted to decide if and when they'd like to get pregnant. Margaret Sanger, a nurse from New York, was one of the biggest crusaders of the birth control movement. In fact, she coined the term 'birth control'. She would dream of a 'magic pill' as easy to take as aspirin that would allow people to plan their families. At this time, doctors were recommending people rinse their vaginas with diluted carbolic acid after having sex to prevent a pregnancy. Yes, literal acid. This practice was called douching, and that's where the word douchebag comes from. Sanger eventually opened her first clinic in Brooklyn, New York in 1916, which was the first step to the Planned Parenthood Foundation. For this she promptly got arrested nine days later. Yes, people have gone to *jail* to allow our free access to contraception.

At the same time, doctors across the world were scrambling to make available other contraceptive options too. Dr Grafenberg, of the G-spot fame, developed one of the world's first intra-uterine devices (IUDs), using some silk wrapped around a silver wire that would be inserted into the uterus. He used German silver, which contained silver, copper, and nickel, which led to the eventual discovery that copper is toxic to sperm. And that is how copper IUDs were born, although the development was quite slow; because World War II was raging at that time! During the Nazi regime, all contraceptive research was stopped because, apparently, that could be a 'threat' to Aryan women.

Thankfully, things went full throttle after the war, and the first pill was approved in the US in 1957, to 'treat severe menstrual disorders'. There was a *warning* on the label which said that taking the pill would have a contraceptive effect, which led to an enthusiastically large number of women in the US suddenly developing 'severe menstrual disorders' and wanting to go on the pill. It took a few more years to make it readily available for everyone across the globe, during which time it was learnt that the original pills contained a seriously heavy dose of hormones., which meant that they caused severe side effects. Because the US had weird laws around contraception, the pill was tested on unsuspecting Puerto Rican women who were not fully made aware of the side effects. This ruined the public's trust in the pill. It did not help that people were afraid women would become so sexually empowered that they would start banging everything left, right, and centre, and it would lead to the ultimate demise of 'good girls'. At this time, there was also a really poorly made IUD called the Dalkon Shield that led to infertility and death in several users. People wanted contraception but they were reasonably confused by all the bad headlines going around. This led to some comically strange at-home contraceptive methods, such as douching your vagina with Coca-Cola. Now, I can tell you for sure that it did not work as a contraceptive. But it certainly gives a whole new meaning to the Coca-Cola tagline, 'taste the feeling'.

Fortunately, this led to a lot of changes. Informative leaflets detailing side effects were included, formulations were improved, hormonal dosages were reduced, and the American singer Loretta Lynn wrote a whole song about the cool pill. We got the copper IUD in 1988, birth control implants in 1991, and emergency contraception in 1993, (coincidentally also the year I was born.) In fact, 1993 was a really cool year for contraception. In 1993, *The Economist* called the pill one of the Seven Wonders of the Modern World, claiming that this was the first time in human history that 'men and women were truly partners'. (Oh, and of course, y'know, me, the star was also born . . . *flips hair and acts cool*). The 2000s saw incredible progress in this field with hormonal IUDs, hormonal rings, birth control patches, more emergency contraception, and improved birth control implants becoming available. We now have researchers working on sprays, gels, baths, and male contraception.

You might wonder why I took you on such a long journey to explain the history of contraceptives. I wanted to highlight to you what a dramatic impact contraceptives have made in our world. I also wanted to draw your attention to the fact that for most of history, people had to get really frikkin inventive if they wanted to avoid children. Although we still have barriers to access contraceptives, it has gotten SO much better. And we need to scream from the rooftops about the impact of contraception. Even today, half of all US pregnancies are unwanted. Studies show that globally, hundreds of millions of women want to use contraception, but they're stopped because of cultural opposition and the fear of side effects. Some estimates show that in India, we could prevent 35,000 maternal deaths and close to 1.2 million infant deaths, if people's contraceptive needs were met. Access to contraception is essential for the well-being of people and society.

In the last 70–90 years, we have seen incredible growth, education, and economic upliftment in the state (and status) of women. Pregnancies interfere with the education of young people—in fact, we have seen more and more women being able to access higher education, and pursue college degrees if they have access to birth control and can practise family planning. For people who could access the pill, college enrolment was higher by 20 per cent in 1970! Not just education, but economics was also impacted. Planned and unplanned pregnancies cost a lot of money; money that is hard to make if you're constantly pregnant. When you give people the choice of when they want to have a kid, it leads to better outcomes for everyone—healthier kids are born to more educated parents. Parents can earn more and provide better for their kids, ensuring fewer children (and adults) are driven into poverty. There is a lesser burden on healthcare, and we have healthier people overall—reproductive autonomy makes the *world* better.

The pill has been a revolution: it's easy to use, it puts the control in your hands, and it comes with a LOT of non-contraceptive benefits. It undoubtedly changed women's lives, allowing us to keep sex and reproduction separate, and control our fertility. As anybody who has heard the dreaded '*beta khushakhabari kab de rahe ho*' from a relative will know, there is way too much interference from other people about what goes on in our uteri. This level of autonomy in women's hands is unprecedented in human history! Of course, some people are going to be alarmed (and very unhappy) at this development. I'm absolutely not saying there are no side effects to the pill. I'm just trying to make sure you see that a lot of the (mostly inaccurate) 'anti-pill' stuff you see on the internet has roots in a more serious problem of misogyny.

The pill is a feminist issue.

19

Contraception

Ek thaa raaja
Ek thii raani
Dono mar gaye
Khatam kahani

[Once there was a king
and a queen
They both died
The end]

—Old Hindi saying

Have you watched *Dilwale Dulhaniya Le Jayenge*? If you haven't, here's a brief intro to the cult favourite Bollywood film. We have Raj and Simran, two very good-looking people who have fallen madly in love and want to spend the rest of their lives together. Then we have Babuji, Simran's dad, who is . . . not on board with this decision (for reasons that have nothing to do with our chapter and so we will skip that part). Why am I telling you about this more than twenty-year-old film for our birth control chapter? To understand contraception, of course. In this analogy, Raj is the sperm, Simran is the egg, and Babuji is the contraception. In our retelling, Babuji will be cartoonishly villainous in his attempts to stop Raj and Simran from being together.

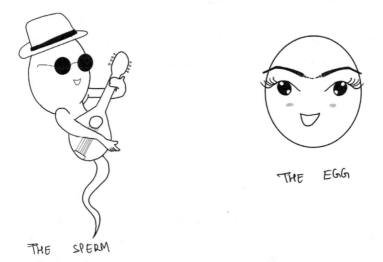

THE   SPERM

THE   EGG

Our story begins in Ovary School, where Simran studies with her other egg friends. Now, Simran is no ordinary egg; she's the smartest, prettiest, and most ambitious egg in Ovary School. She's a superstar egg, destined for huge success, growing bigger and stronger than her other egg friends. Her teachers and parents encourage Simran to go abroad for further studies and *jaa jee le apni zindagi*. Unbeknownst to them, Simran has another motivation to go abroad. Simran is in love with a boy called Raj, who she wants to marry and live with in the faraway Uterus-land.

And so, supported by her friends and family, Simran finally decides to leave her home. (This process is called ovulation—when the egg leaves the ovary, after a huge surge in a hormone called LH.)

After Simran leaves the house, meaning the egg leaves the ovary, one of two things can happen:

1. Simran can meet Raj, fall in love, and live with him forever (egg meets sperm, and makes a baby).
2. Simran can't meet Raj, becomes sad, and cries really hard. There may be some bloodshed involved (egg can't meet sperm, so no baby is made; and you get a period).

In the first scenario:

Simran reaches the faraway foreign lands and runs to meet her lover. After waiting for so long, Raj and Simran are desperate to see each other and err . . . make love. Blinded by hormones and horniness, Raj and Simran decide to elope. So, one night, Raj and Simran meet in this secret, dark, long alleyway (the Fallopian tube) and get married. Deliriously in love, they fuse and become one person, and move to their cosy home in Uterus-land. (And that is how a pregnancy happens—the egg meets sperm inside the Fallopian tube, forms an embryo, and gets implanted inside the thick endometrium of the uterus.)

In the second scenario:

Simran can't meet Raj, and there is a lot of pain and tears. Simran gets very very sad, shrivels up and dies. Obviously, without Raj and Simran, their house in Uterus-land is now useless. So, Uterus-land throws out all their household stuff, in order to make space (hopefully) for a new Raj–Simran couple the following month. (And that's how periods happen. When there is no embryo to implant, the uterus sheds its endometrium, which all comes out as blood and mucus in a period. My mom calls it 'the weeping of a disappointed uterus', which I think is very fitting.)

Thankfully, the second scenario is more common as otherwise our horny asses would be pregnant *all the time*. Like every love marriage in India, we have a *pyaar mein deewaar*— meet Babuji (contraception). Babuji is very protective about his daughter, and will never let her go out to *udao* her romantic *gulchharre*. So, Babuji works in many, many ways to stop Simran from meeting Raj. Some of these ways are as follows:

1. Barrier methods (condoms) and natural methods (withdrawal) = Babuji doesn't let Raj into his city at all. Raj is trapped outside the city walls, and Simran carries on with her life without ever meeting Raj.
2. Hormones (pills, IUDs, injectables, emergency) = Babuji traps Simran in the house, and also keeps Raj outside the city walls. Maybe also destroys their house in Uterus-land, for good measure.
3. Tubectomy and Vasectomy = Babuji orders house arrest for Raj and Simran, never letting either of them out into the real world, trapping them in their homes forever.

Confused? Let's discuss them one by one.

Barrier methods

We have a whole chapter on condoms—external and internal—so I will politely skip this. But there are some other types of barrier contraceptives also available. We have things like diaphragms and cervical caps that cover the cervix, not allowing sperm to enter. Unfortunately, they are not easily available in India, and require special fitting by a doctor, so I'm going to move on.

Hormonal Methods

There is a lot to say about hormonal contraception, so I've dedicated the next chapter to that. Feel free to jump to that if you'd like, and come back and read this afterwards.

Natural Methods

If you'd rather not do anything in terms of putting stuff in your body or take any pills, and you want to let nature take its own course, you can use natural methods for contraception. Bear in mind that often letting nature take its own course involves getting very very pregnant. There are five main methods of natural contraception:

1. Abstinence: Where you just don't have sex. I mean, this is the most surefire way to not get pregnant, right? Abstinence is the *only* form of birth control that is 100 per cent effective.
2. Outercourse: Where you don't insert the penis into the vagina. You can just do all your hanky-panky *uppar uppar*

se, with no insertions. Here, you can do things like oral sex, mutual masturbation (where you both help each other get off), use sex toys, dry hump (grind on top of each other without any genitals directly touching or inserting), or even kiss and make out. Some even consider anal sex as outercourse. These are really great and can really help you connect intimately with your partner; only make sure no semen actually gets near your genitals. Oh, and you can still get sexually transmitted infections this way.

3. Breast feeding: Yepppp . . . when you are breastfeeding (on a very specific schedule, and only and only breastfeeding—no other kind of food for your bubs), your body stops ovulating. If there is no ovulation, meaning no egg is released, then how will Raj and Simran meet if Simran isn't there now? You have to be very specific, only feed your baby breast milk directly from the source, (no pumping, and no extra non-breast milk feed), and it works only for six months. The rules are strict, but if done correctly, lactational amenorrhea, (the technical science-y name for this technique) can be quite effective. Speak with your doctor to discuss this if you are planning to do it.

4. Withdrawal, aka coitus interruptus: This is where the penis is pulled out of the vagina before cumming. This is the technique practised by most people, and has a decently high failure rate. You can get preggo if this is not done perfectly, so make sure to withdraw well in time, so that absolutely no semen leaks into the vagina, and then don't let the semen fall on the vulva. Although unlikely, it can mix with the vaginal secretions and climb up into

the uterus. You're also exposed to STIs with this method; but adding a condom to your withdrawal method not only protects you from the STI risk but also makes your withdrawal so much safer. If you are going to do this, I highly recommend using this technique with a condom.

5. Fertility awareness method (FAM): Well fam, isn't it ironic that the FAM method stops you from having a baby? Sorry that was a rubbish joke. Unlike my joke, FAM can be quite cool. Fertility awareness methods use natural strategies to prevent a pregnancy. There are a lot of ways you can practise FAM but it requires you to (*a*) have regular cycles and (*b*) be diligent with tracking your cycles and symptoms. There are three main ways of doing this: temperature tracking, cycle tracking, and mucus (um yes) tracking.

With temperature tracking, you track your temperature every single day at the same time, right after waking up. Like you can't pee or poop or randomly browse Instagram on your phone, you must take your temperature first. This works because when you are ovulating, your temperature is raised by around one degree. Obviously, this is complicated and can fluctuate. (I mean, you can get a fever! Also, stress, alcohol, etc. can also change your temperature.) You also need to be very rigorous with measuring your temp. But it's a great way to understand and feel more in touch with your body and avoid consuming medicines, if you don't like that.

Then we have cycle tracking, where instead of running your cycle on a track—yes, I know it's a terrible joke—you track your menstrual cycles. After ovulation, if the egg is not fertilized, it takes your body about 14 days to start having a period. So, this means that your ovulation occurs 14 days before your period arrives. This can be a very handy tool to estimate your fertile period using just a calendar. Let's say your period arrived on the 30th of March, then 30 − 14 = 16, so you'd have ovulated around the 16th of March. It would be best to avoid sex up to 5 days before (16 − 5 = 10) and 3 days after (16 + 3 = 19) your ovulation date, i.e., from the 10th to the 19th of March. All other times of the month are safe. This is a fairly easy method, without complicated readings; but it does require your cycles to be really regular! Doing this on an irregular cycle will go badly—like, it will lead to having babies you did not want badly.

And then comes mucus tracking, where you analyse your vaginal discharge to figure out if you are fertile or not. You see, your discharge changes in texture and colour throughout your monthly cycle. Right after your period, you may not notice a lot of discharge. These are the dry and safe days. Later, in the pre-ovulation part of your cycle, your discharge is likely to be yellow/white and sticky. This is also a mostly safe time. When you are most fertile, around the time of your ovulation, this mucus becomes stretchy and clear, like egg white. Obviously, you do not want to be having sex without any additional contraceptives at this time. After ovulation, your mucus becomes thick or disappears altogether. The pre-ovulation and ovulation phases are generally considered fertile, so avoid unprotected sex during those times. This is another great method of really getting in touch with your body, without adding additional hormones. It can be a sticky (lolol) affair though, if you aren't quite comfortably sticking your hands inside yourself and analysing the goo coming out of you (ooh that rhymes!).

Surgery

But what if you're just like, so done with this whole idea of baby prevention that you want to put a lock on your baby-making factory? Babies banned forever! Well, lucky for you, you actually can do that! Let's talk about permanent contraception.

So, depending on who gets it, permanent contraception can be of two types: tubectomy, (where the person with the uterus gets the surgery) or vasectomy (where the person with the penis gets the surgery).

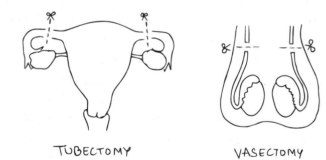

TUBECTOMY   VASECTOMY

In a tubectomy, we simply tie up or cut off a part of the Fallopian tubes. With this part cut, the place where the egg meets the sperm is gone. So, the egg that is ovulated every month essentially floats about in the pelvis like an *awaara* egg, until it dies, and the sperm also has nobody to meet. It's a quick and simple surgery, but is quite invasive as it involves cutting into the body and going all the way inside the pelvis to cut the tubes. You need anaesthesia, and a whole ass surgical procedure.

A vasectomy on the other hand is much simpler, where we tie and cut off a part of the vas deferens. What is the vas though? Sperm is made inside the testicles (sperm production factories) and they leave the testicles to join the penis using a special tube called the vas deferens. Consider it the super-highway of the male reproductive system. If you were to cut the vas deferens, there'd be no effect on the sperm production, but they just wouldn't be able to exit the body via the penis at the time of ejaculation. Since semen (the fluid) is not made in the testicles, and is added along the way, there is no effect on semen production. The semen is still made and it still comes out, but it contains no sperm. It's a bit like pulp-free juice. Think of it as the king ordering Anarkali to be buried alive in the wall in *Mughal-e-Azam*. Well here, instead of Anarkali, our Saleem Sperm is *chunawao*-ed alive inside the *deewaar*. The sperm can never leave the testicles, and never meet his *dilruba*, the egg. With this, our sperm and egg die, and this brings us to the end of our permanent contraceptive methods.

And if you want something less invasive, cheaper, and easier to use? Well, we have condoms, of course!

20

Condoms

Meet the condom. Aka *chhatri*, love glove, raincoat, rubber, cundome . . . basically whatever you want to call it. It's usually a thin piece of latex that, again usually, covers the penis and protects you from unwanted pregnancies and STIs. In fact, it is the only contraceptive in the world that protects you from STIs. Condoms are a 'barrier' contraceptive, meaning they form a barrier between your body and your partner's body fluids, which carry baby-making sperms and maybe STIs. The condom is very very wonderful, and very very underappreciated.

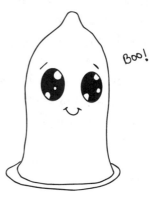

There is so much to learn about condoms: for example, did you know that condoms are related to the tyres in your car? Sounds weird, but it's super interesting. You see, most commonly, condoms are made of latex. Latex is essentially rubber + water. Now rubber is also a very interesting material, but traditionally it wasn't as um . . . rubbery . . . as its modern-day variant. For most of history, rubber was thick and inflexible, until Mr Charles Goodyear discovered vulcanization. Yes, the same Mr Goodyear from the Goodyear tyres. Vulcanization is the process by which rubber is made flexible, leading it to become soft, thin, and bendy. All of these properties are extremely important, especially for condoms, because nobody likes thick, rough, and hard condoms. Before vulcanized rubber was available, condoms were thick and only covered the top of the penis, (like a hat). In fact, early condoms were called capotes or bonnets, or even American caps. Apparently, even Casanova, the most famous lover in the world, was said to use them. Yay to Mr Goodyear for unexpectedly changing the world. (What a great example of how a passion for solving problems in your field can have such far-reaching effects. I will get off my preachy motivational train now. Bet you did not expect that in a chapter on condoms, did you?) Anyway, Tyreman did some cool shit with rubber and we developed latex and made condoms out of them.

While latex can be natural or synthetic, condoms are mostly made of natural latex. Some rubbery sap oozes out of trees, which is then collected, processed, and made into latex. Some people are allergic to latex (around 4 per cent of the world population), for whom we also have latex-free condoms made from polyurethane and polyisoprene. For the more crunchy granola types, we even have all-natural hippie condoms made out of animal intestines! These are interestingly called lambskin condoms, even though there is no actual lambskin in them. They're more expensive than regular condoms, and have tiny holes in them through which bacteria and viruses can pass through, although sperm can't, so they're not recommended for protection against STIs.

Other than the classic fit-on-top-of-the-penis, we also have another type of condom which can be inserted internally. The so-called 'female condom' or 'internal condom' can be put inside the vagina or the anus and serves the same purpose as a regular condom. (Although they can be a bit clunky, some people really enjoy using them.) They come with the huge advantage that they can be inserted a few hours before sex, which eliminates the awkward fumbling around for a condom (or ignoring the condom entirely) that can happen in the middle of a hot and heavy session. It also provides more agency to the person who is using them if their partner refuses to wear one. Internal condoms can help save time and protect your bodily autonomy, which is a win in my books because condom use is really important. Dude, condoms save lives—no matter what kind you use.

This is not me being extra. Condoms are really effective; they are 98 per cent effective in preventing a pregnancy, if used correctly. Compare that with the pull-out method, where your partner pulls out their penis just before ejaculating. Sounding like it comes straight out of a Harry Potter novel, this process is called coitus interruptus, and has a pregnancy prevention rate as low as 70 per cent. Not only do condoms protect you from accidentally making babies when you don't want them, but they also protect you from STIs. Regular condom use lowers your risk of Hepatitis B, gonorrhoea, and chlamydia by up to 90 per cent. As anyone who has lived through the AIDS panic of the 1980s will tell you, condoms are very effective in protecting you from HIV, the infection that can lead to

AIDS. There is an 80–95 per cent lower risk of contracting HIV if you use condoms. Using a condom makes sex 10,000 times (yes, ten THOUSAND times) safer when it comes to contracting HIV. I mean, at this point, it just sounds like a no-brainer. Everyone should use condoms. All the time. (Unless of course you are trying to get pregnant.)

Which brings me to a very interesting fact about condoms or using condoms when trying to get pregnant. Wait, what? Don't condoms prevent a pregnancy? Why would you need to use them when you're trying to do the baby-making thing? Well . . . you see, the Church doesn't approve of the use of contraceptives. Of any kind. Oh, and no masturbation too. According to the church, sex is meant for a man and a woman, who are joined together in marriage, to make babies. This is all well and fine (I don't agree with this, but I will keep my opinion aside for now) for most people, except it really becomes a problem for people who are trying to get pregnant and having trouble. If you were having difficulty conceiving, you would go to a doctor who will run some tests—testing your and your partner's hormones, as well as testing the quality of your semen. This usually involves you going to a quiet room and jacking off into a plastic cup, and handing it to your doctor for studying. This is called a semen analysis, and it's a very regular and important test in fertility investigations.

But remember that whole thing about the church being against masturbation? Yeah, well, that clearly creates a problem with the whole producing a semen sample by masturbating thing. So, people came up with a nifty solution. Instead of masturbating, how about you just bang your partner wearing a condom, ejaculate into it, and use that condom like a collection bag for your semen. This way, you are having sex in your marriage for the purpose of procreation. Sounds perfect? Well, almost. There is one more problem left. You see, condoms are a contraceptive method, and as we know, the church does not approve of them. So, now what? Do we look for a new loophole? Well thankfully, doctors being smart *and* sneaky found a new way out of the problem—how about making a small hole in the condom? That way, it still works as a collection bag without being a contraceptive, and there is no masturbation involved. Yay *jugaad*! And that, my friends, is the story of how condoms are used by religious couples who want to go through fertility treatments without any problems in the god department. The Holy Condom or the Holey Condom? You decide.

Apart from God-approved fertility treatments though, holes in your condoms are not a good idea. You see, condoms work by shielding you from your partner's body fluids. At the top end of a condom, there is a small space, called a teat, where semen collects. Always remember to squeeze this teat when putting a condom on. This way, that space isn't filled up by your penis, so that when you ejaculate into it, all your semen collects over here instead of rolling out all over the penis and exiting your condom. A hole in there would kinda make this whole latex penis burrito useless. Thankfully, condoms are tested very rigorously: manufacturers run an electric current through every single condom that's made to ensure it is intact (the physics of which I don't quite understand, but luckily, I am just a doctor and not a physicist, so we will conveniently skip this part). They are stretched and inspected from every corner to keep things neat. (This part is extremely fascinating.

For example, did you know that a condom can be stretched up to 800 times its original length? Tell that to the next guy who says they're 'too big' to fit into a condom. And that a condom can hold up to 3 litres of fluid? Although, I sincerely hope you are not producing that much jizz, or you need an urgent trip to the doctor.) Sometimes, whole batches of condoms are run through surprise checks to make sure it all stays nifty. To keep things even more safe, condoms also come with an expiration date. Each condom lasts anywhere between one to five years, so maybe that condom you bought on a date during college that has been sitting in your wallet still may not be the best thing to use anymore.

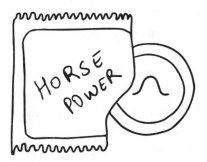

Other than expiring, there is another huge (or tiny) reason why your condom can fail— the sensitive size situation. Some people like to boast about having an absolutely monster penis (even though that makes no difference to how much sexual pleasure your partner feels, it's full *bakwas*) and therefore, requiring massive condoms. But if you're lying, and you buy an extra-large condom for an average-size penis, there is a very high risk of the condom slipping off mid-act and failing. Similarly, a small condom on a large penis can tear if it is too tight. Basically, just like you should buy shoes the right size for your feet, otherwise they will hurt, you should also buy condoms the right size for your penis. (Oh, and contrary to the popular idea, your shoe size has nothing to do with your penis size. Sorry to the fans of Joey Tribbiani.) Wearing two condoms also does not make it more effective in preventing a pregnancy than wearing one condom. In fact, two condoms can slip off or tear more easily. Wear one, correct-size condom and dispose of it after use. It's really quite simple.

Oh no, wait, sorry, I forgot one very important point in this simple condom use strategy—other than ripping and slipping, condoms can also break down and degrade when they come in contact with oils. This means that you should NOT be using Vaseline or some random kitchen oil as a lubricant when using a condom. If you want to use a lubricant—and you should, because yay lubes—with your condom, stick to simple water-based lubricants. You can purchase these in offline or online stores, and they cost anywhere between Rs 100 to Rs 2000. Leave the olive oil for seasoning your salad.

And since we're talking about food—what's up with strawberry-flavoured condoms?! Or vanilla, chocolate, mango milkshake, paan, or whatever the hell flavour—what's the point? Penises and vaginas don't have taste buds, so why are we adding flavour to condoms? Does it add to the ambience? Well, as it turns out, oral sex is surprisingly good at spreading STIs and you should totally be using condoms over the penis when going down on it. *That's* why condoms are flavoured (apparently rubber-scented latex covered dick is not a popular candy flavour). And not just for penises, you should also cover the vulva or anus if you're going down on someone. But um, how exactly does a condom fit over a vulva?

Well, it doesn't, and that's why you need dental dams. This might leave you feeling very confused if you're a dentist, but bear with me. Dental dams were invented by dentists to keep your teeth away from saliva when performing dental surgery. Someone in history found out another cool use for them, where you use dental dams (which are essentially a square of latex) to cover genitals in order to have safe oral sex. Cunnilingus (or eating pussy) can also transmit STIs through body fluids, and covering the genitals, so there is no direct contact between the genitals (+ genital fluids) and the mouth, can help us overcome this problem. Unfortunately, dental dams are either not easily available in the market or when available are stupidly expensive. Fortunately, you can make your own dental dam at home and keep yourself safe! Yay! Simply take a condom, and cut off its head like Marie Antoinette. This will leave you with a condom tube. Slice through one side of this tube, and you will have a square piece of latex—tada! Here's your dental dam! You can also use some clear plastic wrap if you're in a pinch. (But this is not as reliable because plastic wrap often contains teeny, tiny holes to let steam escape. Teeny, tiny holes that are big enough to also let STI-causing bacteria and viruses escape.) Basically, please make sure there is some barrier to protect you from these direct body fluids.

Some people complain that using dental dams and condoms for any kind of sex can reduce pleasure. But honestly, wouldn't feeling safe make things more pleasurable? If that sounds like bullshit to you (hey you're not a sex education nerd like me), you can make condoms a part of foreplay—instead of pausing and fumbling around awkwardly to put it on, engage your partner in rolling the condom or dam on you. This can be sexy, exciting, and a huge turn on! Plus, now we have safety, my guys. Condoms can be foreplay! In the meantime, we also have researchers working on spray-on condoms and 'invisible' condoms. (The Bill & Melinda Gates Foundation promises $1 million to creative entrepreneurs who can invent the 'next generation' condom that enhances pleasure so that more people are encouraged to use them!)

Other than being flavoured for oral sex, the humble, versatile condom comes in another type: textured. Ribbed, dotted, rib and dotted . . . there are many textured varieties that claim to enhance sexual pleasure when used during penetration. If you like using them, well and good. They can add friction and be exciting. But there are two things to remember when using these fancy condoms.

No. 1. Most people with a vagina orgasm from the stimulation of the clitoris. Adding textures during penetration can be really exciting, but it will not lead to some magical vaginal orgasm benefits.

No. 2. USE LUBE. As friction increases, your likelihood of getting vaginal irritation also increases, which can mean sensitivity, pain, and even infections. This is especially important for anal sex, as the anus does not have its own natural lubrication factory like the vagina does. Lubricant can help counteract all these side effects, while still letting you enjoy the texture.

While textured condoms are made for the benefit of women, men have specific climax-delay condoms designed for them. They contain a mild numbing or anaesthetic agent, which is supposed to help people who have an orgasm too quickly. I personally am against such condoms, because there are a lot of other more effective techniques that can help you delay orgasms. Instead of, you know, numbing your knob. I mean, how are you supposed to enjoy sex if your dick is numb? Not just that, but it can also cause irritation and rashes on your penis. Sounds like a big fat 'nope' to me. Historically, some condoms also had a spermicide (a chemical that kills sperm) called nonoxynol coating to *really* protect you from a pregnancy. Unfortunately, they were found to be irritating to the vagina, and also increased the risk of UTIs and HIV. They were stopped very quickly after. For some people with more singular tastes, we also have novelty glow-in-the-dark condoms. A new kind of lightsaber, if you will.

But condoms are not just for protecting the weapon in your pants; some people have also used condoms to protect another kind of weapon: rifles. Yes. Really. Since World War II, condoms have been used by nifty soldiers to protect the front end of the gun from sand, muck, and dirt. Creatively called 'camouflage condoms', they can be rolled up over the snout of the rifle to make it waterproof and dust proof. On the other end of the spectrum, smugglers have long used condoms to secretly transport drugs by filling them up with the contraband and either swallowing them or sticking them up their butts. This can get dangerous very quickly, as condoms can burst, release the drugs, and cause death by overdose. On a lighter note, condoms can also be used to cover microphones to fashion makeshift underwater mics or hydrophones (real hydrophones are pretty expensive, and condoms are . . . not). And, of course, if you ever get a vaginal ultrasound, you will see your doctor roll up a simple, lubricated condom over the ultrasound probe before penetrating (ahem) you with it.

However, you cover your junk, please do cover your junk. And not just for show—use the condom for the duration of the entire sexual act. This might seem strange as a suggestion, but there is a form of sexual abuse called stealthing. Stealthing is when someone secretly removes a condom in the middle of sex, without the consent of the other person involved. It is a form of sexual assault, and some countries such as the UK and Germany have made this a criminal act. Misleading your partner into believing that they are safe from pregnancy and STIs, and then breaching that trust is just not okay. Some people recognize this as a form of rape. Don't stealth, okay? We've been a seriously sex-positive nation through history, and you should carry that reputation with honour and pride.

No, seriously. India was one of the first few countries in *the world* to establish a family planning programme, all the way back in 1952. Condoms were introduced to the country in the 1940s, when they would be imported from abroad. This was obviously ridiculously expensive; so in the early 1960s, the Indian government set up Hindustan Latex Limited in the rubber-rich state of Kerala to support the National Family Planning Programme and made our own *swadesi* condoms. And thus, Nirodh (meaning protection, literally) was born. Funnily, Nirodh was originally meant to be called Kamaraj (after Kamadev, the Hindu god of carnal love), but that name was quickly dropped after the makers realized that the President of the Indian National Congress was a certain Mr K. Kamaraj. Nevertheless, we have grown from there to a Rs 1500 crore market for condoms over the years.

This is probably the longest chapter in the whole book, so I hope you get the message that I have been trying to drill into your head using the last three thousand words: using condoms regularly can be one of the BEST things you can do for your sexual health. Just use them? It's literally the most *sasta* and *tikau* safety precaution out there. As my hero Dr Jen Gunter says, condoms are vagina superheroes. Plus, isn't it like a tiny raincoat for your penis? That's hella cute.

21

Hormonal Contraception

How horrific are hormones! Or, at least, that's what a lot of 'health coaches' on Instagram want you to believe. In reality, hormones are actually pretty chill and useful. They're just chemicals made by your body to coordinate its different functions and help your body machinery run smoothly. One of the *many* things your hormones do is prepare your body for sex and pregnancy, using two main hormones called estrogen and progesterone. They are secreted in different amounts throughout your menstrual cycle to help develop and release an egg, help that egg meet the sperm, implant inside the uterus, or shed the lining of the uterus in case the sperm and egg don't meet. Without the correct doses of these hormones at the right time, our species might not even exist!

Since they're obviously so hugely impactful on the, y'know, continued existence of our species on this planet, it was very important and useful to understand them. And so, scientists got to work on making synthetic versions of these hormones so we could control how and when we made babies. Pretty important stuff. The first hormonal contraceptive was a pill called Enovid, which was released in 1956. Although initially meant to 'regulate menstruation', it had an interesting and very enjoyable 'side effect' of preventing pregnancies. It was a smashing success! You could just ask your doctor to 'regulate menstruation', take a pill, and have as much sex as you'd like without worrying about screaming babies. While the early hormone pills did work pretty effectively (even as a side effect) at the baby controlling end of things, unfortunately, they had very high doses of hormones that came with pretty severe side effects. And we are talking about real side effects this time; not fun ones like accidentally having the superpower of not getting pregnant and having to put your entire life on hold, y'know.

Aside from the hormone overdose, there were also some very nasty human rights violations in the testing of these drugs. It was noted that the earliest developers of birth control pills had their ideas for contraception rooted in racism (definitely something worth reading up on later). The racist foundations, coupled with human rights issues, and of course the plethora of side effects from the super high hormones left a lingering impact on the legacy of hormonal pills. Even though the pill has been recognized as one of the biggest contributors to women's liberation and feminism, birth control pills started with a bad reputation and never quite recovered.

But my ideological, social, and historical rant aside (because we have a whole chapter on it lol), let's talk about how hormones actually work in preventing a pregnancy. To begin with, we need to establish that we have many different methods of hormonal contraception, not just the pill. The journey that started with the pill has now led to the development of many different kinds of hormonal contraception. We have a huge variety ranging from pills, patches, and rings, all the way to implants and devices that can be inserted inside you and which last for years. One of the simplest ways of understanding the many different types is by figuring out how often you are willing to put in the effort for contraception:

-   If you are okay making a daily effort, you can be on hormonal birth control pills.
-   If you'd prefer something weekly, you can get hormonal patches that need to be changed every week.
-   If you'd rather only remember your contraception duties every month, you can use the hormonal ring.
-   If you like to go to the doctor every three months, you can get an injectable hormonal contraceptive.
-   Or you can go for long-acting reversible contraception (LARC), which can be taken every 4 years with hormonal implants; or every 3–12 years, with an IUD.

This may feel a bit overwhelming, so we're going to break them down one by one. We'll also talk a little bit about the negative PR surrounding some of these methods, understand the science behind them, and address common concerns. Beginning with the contraceptive pill, let's go back to Simran, Raj, and Babuji to understand this.

Birth control pills, or oral contraceptive pills, are a kind of hormone-containing medicines that provide contraception. Depending on the hormone combination in them, there are two kinds of contraceptive pills: combined oral contraceptive pills and progestin-only pills. Combined oral contraceptive pills contain both estrogen and progestin (a synthetic progesterone) that work together to help prevent a pregnancy. They work in two ways: (1) by stopping ovulation, i.e., preventing the egg release from the ovary, or not allowing Simran to leave the house, and (2) by secreting a thick mucus at the entrance of the uterus, so sperm gets trapped and can't get into the uterus, or not allowing Raj inside the city walls. With no egg released, and the sperm being unable to enter the uterus, a pregnancy cannot happen. Babuji is successful! Progestin-only pills, on the other hand, work by making the mucus thick, so sperm can't get in, i.e., Raj is banned from entering, and by thinning the endometrium, which is the inside lining of the uterus, so even if the egg and sperm meet, the pregnancy cannot stay and develop inside the uterus, destroying Raj and Simran's future home. And Babuji is once again successful!

So, while it's a bit more complicated, essentially all birth control pills work in three main ways: preventing ovulation, making the mucus thicker, and sometimes changing the endometrium. This way, the sperm and the egg are not allowed to meet, and on the off chance they do meet, they are not allowed to implant inside the uterus. They come in different packs, but usually involve having the same pill every day for 21 or 28 days. Some contain 21-day active pills, and 7 days of placebo pills, (which don't contain any active hormone but are there just to keep you in the habit of consuming a pill every day) or iron pills (to help supplement the blood loss you will have on your period). We even have some special pills which, although currently not available in India, can be taken for 84 days in a row, with a 7-day break. This way you only get your period four times in a year!

No matter what type and regimen you use, you should start your pills in the first five days of your cycle. Your cycle begins on the first day of your period. So, if you got your period today, you would start counting from today, and this would be Day One. Your doctor will advise you more specifically on when to start though. Pills can also be used for all kinds of other non-contraceptive benefits, such as reducing heavy and painful periods, acne, as well as other conditions like endometriosis, adenomyosis, and PCOS. Like all medications, they come with risks and side effects. Usually, we avoid prescribing the pill if you have a history of high blood pressure, clotting issues, are a smoker, or have migraines. Side effects include tender breasts, nausea, spotting, headaches, and bloating. Some people may report an increase in libido, whereas some may report a decrease—our sex drive continues to befuddle us. While there is a lot more to the pill, including problems, myths, and misconceptions, we will discuss them in detail in another chapter.

Now, let's move on to other options like patches, which we don't have in India (*KLPD ho gaya*). They're the same thing as pills, except instead of swallowing them, you put them on your body like a sticker. You change it every week for three weeks, after which you go a patch-free week, when you get your period. Alternatively, you can also get a vaginal ring, which goes inside your vagina and lasts three weeks. After three weeks, you go for a ring-free week when you get your period, and then put a new ring in after. Side effects are similar, but you don't have to remember to take daily pills. Sounds great but remember this you will not get in India, so please don't get excited.

Now that I've done some getting-you-excited-for-no-reason *waali bakwas*, I'll offer you a more legitimate (and even longer lasting) option: the injectable contraceptive. The chemical compound (which actually has a very long ass name) is called DMPA, so we *desis* very cutely call it Dimpa, or (less cutely) Depo-Provera. It contains a progestin hormone and basically works by keeping Simran in by suppressing ovulation and by keeping Raj out by thickening cervical mucus to prevent sperm from going in. You can go to your doctor and get injections every twelve weeks, so you can go without worrying about contraception for three months! Like other hormonal contraceptives, it reduces your risk of endometrial cancer, painful periods, ovulation pain, and iron-deficiency anaemia; plus it also reduces your risk of pelvic inflammatory disease, ectopic pregnancy, functional ovarian cysts, and fibroids. It can also be very helpful for people with endometriosis. Sounds pretty kickass, and it is! However, it's not recommended to be used for a very long time continuously because of a few significant side effects. Of all the available contraceptives, with DMPA it takes the longest for your fertility to return to normal after stopping use. It can take up to one year! Additionally, this is the only contraceptive that has conclusively been shown to be linked with weight gain. You can speak with your doctor and see if this is a good option for you, because it is for a lot of people. Plus, the added convenience on top is a cherry on the contraceptive cake.

LARC

LARCs, or long-acting reversible contraceptives are contraceptives that can be used for a long term and are reversible. Okay, sorry I'll stop trolling and explain better.

LARCs are the most effective form of birth control because you don't have to remember to take a pill or change your patch every day or every few days. Essentially, they are like a super low-maintenance partner. You put them in and forget about them until you are ready to get pregnant or when they hit expiry. They protect you from a pregnancy for long periods, anywhere from four to twelve years, and are inserted into your body by a trained medical professional. There are two main types: implants and IUDs.

Implants are small plastic rods, about the length of your thumb, that are inserted into your upper arm using a tiny cut. Once in, they release a small amount of progestin into your body for a long period of time, around five years, and stop you from getting pregnant. Same Simran in, Raj out story. It's 99 per cent effective, and if you do decide to get pregnant while yours is still functional, you can just ask your doctor to take it out. Similar side effects as in other hormones for birth control are to be expected, although some people do experience heavier or alternatively lighter periods too. It's a little more expensive, and you may struggle to find it in India.

Aside from getting a contraceptive inside your arm, you could also attack the home base and just get one inside your uterus. These are tiny T-shaped things called IUDs, which basically sit inside your uterus and help prevent a pregnancy. You can get a *non-hormonal* copper IUD (which works because copper is hella toxic to sperm) or *hormonal* IUDs containing progestin (which work by doing the same Simran in, Raj out thing with no ovulation and thick cervical mucus). Copper IUDs can also irritate the endometrium so no implantation occurs, which can lead to the side effects of very heavy, painful periods in some people. Hormonal IUDs, on the other hand, can thin down the endometrium to prevent implantation. This can decrease or almost stop your periods and cramps; and so hormonal IUDs can also be used for people with bad period pain, endometriosis, fibroids, and PCOS.

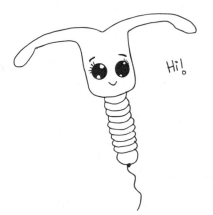

Copper IUDs can also be used as emergency contraception, and they are very effective! The insertion can be painful for some people, so you could take a preventative pain killer before your appointment. Some doctors also offer local anaesthetic on your cervix before inserting the IUD, to avoid any chances of pain. With that said, IUDs are not supposed to be painful for most people. I haven't had one so I wouldn't be able to tell you how it feels, but *most* of my patients say it feels like a pinch. The biggest advantage of an IUD, however, is the fact that they last really long—up to twelve years! So, you can get one in and forget about your uterus and babies for a long, long time. Oh, and if you suddenly want to remember your uterus and babies, you can always ask the doctor to take it out and just like that your fertility is restored. IUDs are mega cool.

Emergency Contraception

IUDs can also be used as emergency contraception when you haven't used any contraceptive method, or your method has failed, and now you're at the risk of getting pregnant. Copper IUDs can be inserted up to five days after the 'risky event' and they can stop a fertilized egg from sticking inside your uterus.

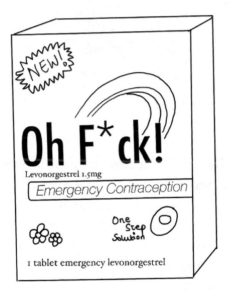

Other than the IUDs, you can also use emergency contraception pills. To be very honest, we're not a 100 per cent sure on how they work, but we think they work mainly by delaying or stopping ovulation, i.e., Simran doesn't get to leave the house at all. You're supposed to consume one within 72 hours of unprotected sex, and they're considered 98 per cent effective. General side effects are nausea, headache, and a change in your period date. Emergency contraceptives are safe to take and do not leave a long-term impact on your fertility. Please don't use them as regular contraceptives though, you have a whole section's worth of contraceptive information now to choose from.

22

Are Birth Control Pills Bad for You?

In the last few chapters, we've learnt a lot about birth control. And I'm sure, even now, many questions remain in your mind. So, let's address the ten most common questions about birth control. I want to keep this section easy for you to read, so you can find clear, direct answers to common myths and misconceptions about the pill here. I hope you won't have withdrawal symptoms from my sparkling wit and awful humour, but this section will have less historical anecdotes and fun facts. Let's begin!

Why do doctors always give hormonal birth control to patients with PCOS (polycystic ovarian syndrome)? Why don't they treat the root cause?

-   The root cause of PCOS is a hormonal imbalance. How do you treat a hormonal imbalance? By balancing the hormones. One of the ways of balancing hormones is using hormonal pills. It's like, if you have an iron deficiency, you can either eat a fuckton of spinach and increase your iron reserves, or you can supplement with iron tablets. One of these methods is not better than the other. We never go and say 'why don't you treat the root cause' to someone who is suffering from a nutrient deficiency of iron in their blood. So why do we say this to people with PCOS? The effectiveness of the method depends on a lot of factors, and for *many* people, the pill works more effectively than just taking lifestyle measures alone.

- More importantly, the hormonal imbalance from PCOS (excess estrogen) can lead to an increased risk of endometrial cancer. Since birth control pills treat the hormonal imbalance and reduce this increased level of estrogen, it reduces your risk of endometrial cancer in the long run. Think of it like how sunscreen protects you from skin cancer in the long run. Someone can definitely come and say, why don't you treat the root cause of sunburns and skin cancer instead of using sunscreen. But that's stupid because using sunscreen *is* protecting you from sun damage, which can lead to skin cancer in the long run.

Do pills increase your risk of getting cancer?

- Hormonal pills reduce your risk of endometrial cancer by 50 per cent, and of ovarian cancer by 25 per cent.
- Since ovarian cancer is often diagnosed very late, people who are at a high risk of getting ovarian cancer could be given pills to help reduce their risk.
- Irregular cycles increase your risk of endometrial cancer. Having regular cycles, even with birth control, reduces your risk of endometrial cancer.
- There is a very small increase in the risk of breast cancer when using pills.

Will having oral contraceptive pills make me infertile?

-   Nope. We have more than enough evidence to show birth
    control pills do not cause infertility, and your fertility
    returns to normal after you stop using the pill.
-   With Depo-Provera injectable contraceptive, it may take
    up to 12 months for your fertility to return to normal.

Do oral contraceptives make me gain weight?

-   So far, we do not have any evidence to show that the
    newer generations of pills cause any weight gain.
-   As we grow older, we normally tend to gain weight
    anyway. That natural weight gain is often incorrectly
    linked with the pill.
-   Depo-Provera injectable contraceptive is the only
    contraceptive that has shown a legitimate link with
    increase in weight.

Will having hormonal pills give me depression?

-   So, a huge Danish study (studying over 1 million people)
    did find a small, but noticeable increase in the risk of
    depression for people who were on hormonal pills.
-   It's also important to note that the increase in risk of
    depression with hormonal pills is quite small: according
    to the study, people who did not take pills had a 1.7 per
    cent risk of being diagnosed with depression. People who
    took the pill had a 2.1 per cent risk. That's just a 0.4 per
    cent increased risk.

- Progesterone-only methods may increase your risk of depression.
- At the end of the day, if something is impacting your mental health, you are the best judge of it, you don't need any numbers and studies. It's best to communicate with your doctor and find an alternative.

Are pills only used for contraception?

- Nope, a lot of people who use birth control don't do it for birth control reasons. Hormonal pills can be very useful for people with acne, painful conditions like endometriosis and adenomyosis, people who have hormonal issues other than PCOS, for people with PCOS, for excessive body hair, for trans women who need the hormones externally, for people with very painful or very heavy menstrual periods, for severe premenstrual syndrome (PMS) and premenstrual dysphoric disorder (PMDD), and for people who have an increased risk of ovarian or endometrial cancer.

Do pills increase the risk of blood clots?

- Directly, yes. Estrogen-containing pills do increase your risk of blood clots. But the risk of blood clots from pregnancy is even higher by several times. Since pills protect you from a pregnancy, they are technically lowering your relative risk of blood clots.
- Overall, pregnancy can be a dangerous health event, and birth control pills (even with their side effects) help reduce that risky event from happening in the first place.

- The side effects and risks that are increased by consuming birth control pills are increased by several times if you are pregnant.
- We'll understand it with an example, with completely *imaginary* numbers: Let's say your baseline risk of getting a clot in your bloodstream is 1 per cent. If you add birth control pills, your risk goes up to 4 per cent. Yes, that is definitely an increase in your risk of getting clots . . . but, if you get pregnant (which birth control pills will stop from happening), your risk of getting clots goes up to 40 per cent. So, with a 4 per cent increase in risk of clots, you are protecting yourself from a 40 per cent increase in risk of clots. Please remember I'm using random hypothetical numbers pulled out of my ass here for ease of explaining; these are not the actual stats.
- This way, birth control pills reduce the relative risk of many conditions that you'd be at a highly increased risk of, if you were to get pregnant.

Do I need a break from birth control?

- Nope. This is a commonly touted claim by hormone coaches and 'natural' healers. Please remember that everything natural is not necessarily good: Tornadoes are natural. But we have no evidence to suggest that birth control breaks are necessary or even required.
- The reason why we have a one-week pill-free time, so you can get your period, is because Dr John Rock, the doctor who conducted the first trials of the pill, was a devout Catholic. The Church doesn't approve of any contraceptive

methods, so Dr Rock claimed that using the pill was a 'natural' method of contraception since it used hormones that naturally occur in the body anyway. This would just act as an extension of the rhythm method or calendar method, by prolonging the post-ovulation period of the cycle. And that's why we have a 'three-week active pill, one-week break' cycle with birth control pills. We don't have any biological reason for why we follow this routine.

These are the science-backed answers to your common questions about birth control pills. I hope this will enable you to use this information wisely when making a decision for your life and your body, instead of falling for ridiculous fear mongering and misinterpreted science.

But *picture abhi baaki hai mere dost*. We cannot end this discussion without talking about the joint responsibility of contraception, or the lack thereof. Condoms are a super user friendly, cheap, highly reversible mode of contraception, that also protect you from STIs, yet hormonal methods of birth control that the woman has to take and is responsible for are far more common. Vasectomies are easier, safer, quicker, less invasive, and more successfully reversible, yet tubectomies are performed far more than vasectomies are. Why this gender disparity in the bedroom? Why do most contraceptives cater to women, when technically they can only get pregnant a few times in a month? Men, on the other hand, are fertile factories, walking around and potentially impregnating hundreds of people every month with their super swimmers! Shouldn't men be the ones who bear the responsibility of contraception?

23

Male Birth Control Pills

Men and their sperm are a little bit like AK-47 guns—always full of sperm, ready to fire with alarming enthusiasm. Every single ejaculate consists of hundreds of millions of sperm, so they have the potential to make someone pregnant at any given hour of any given day. Whereas women ovulate only once a month, and it takes a special full moon night with cosmic rays filtering in from Jupiter to make them pregnant (in case you didn't realize, *I am joking*). Then why are most birth control options aimed at women, with condoms and vasectomies being the only options for men? Why is the responsibility of contraception not shared? Why can't we develop birth control options for men?

Feeling frustrated with these fuckall limited options is natural, there *should* be more money funnelled into male birth control. There should be more options. Not just because the sole duty of contraception should not lie with uterus owners, but also because penis owners deserve choices too. It doesn't help that a lot of penis owners refuse to share the burden of contraception. I mean, condoms are such a cheap and easy solution to the problem but a lot of men refuse to use them saying 'I just don't get that feeling *yaar*' without realizing that if an unwanted pregnancy develops then you'll get many more feelings than you bargained for. Women *toh* can have an emergency contraceptive pill next day anyway *na* . . . why bother with condoms. If men desire long-term contraception, they can always get a vasectomy, but fears about post-surgery pain (and some myths about losing masculinity after surgery) stops them there too. Although I am very thankful that birth control is largely in the hands of women—so men cannot interfere or subjugate women in their reproductive choices, as some of them tend to do—it is truly unfair that the whole burden of planning, purchasing, and dealing with the consequences lies on the woman. And it is also truly unfair that the men do not get a say. But why is it so difficult to make a male birth control pill? How do we empower men with contraceptive choices, and how do we hold them responsible for sharing contraceptive duties? Why haven't we been able to make a male birth control pill for so long?

To understand that let's understand how pregnancy works. Every month, several eggs mature in the ovaries; out of these eggs one becomes the biggest and strongest. This one egg is released at some point during the month in the process we call ovulation, while the rest of the eggs die. This egg stays alive for about 24 hours, during which it must be fertilized. If that doesn't happen, then within 14 days of releasing the egg, you get a period, and your body starts recruiting and developing a fresh new lot of eggs for the next month. Now on the other side, about 200 million sperm are released in every ejaculate, no matter what time of the month the ejaculation happens. (Remember, sperm is prepared fresh every day; testicles make around 1500 sperm *every second*. And ovaries are born with all the eggs they will ever have; you only have about half a million remaining by the time you hit puberty.) So, while a woman can only get pregnant for a few days in a month, men can go around impregnating hundreds of people every single day. In theory, I mean, it's pretty hard to have sex with hundreds of people every day. You'd need some weirdo to calculate how many people you can realistically have sex with in one day to figure out how many you can impregnate.

Don't worry, I am that weirdo, and I calculated. In a 24-hour day, there are about 14 hours available to have sex. I accounted for 8 hours of sleep, and 2 hours of grooming, eating, and preparing for sex. Now the average duration of penetrative sex is about 2–7 minutes, so if we were to take a rough number of 5 minutes per penetrative sexual intercourse, plus at least 30 minutes of refractory period between the sex episodes, one can ejaculate every 35 minutes. That works out to: $14 \times 60 = 840$ minutes, so in the 840 minutes available per day for ejaculation; $840/35 = 24$, one can jizz about 24 times. Obviously, I am not counting for the logistics involved in this such as setting up the vaginas to ejaculate into, the wooing and the foreplay, and the dilution of semen which would happen with so many back-to-back jizzaculations.

ANYWAY, so yeah, penis owners can make about 24 people pregnant daily, which is 720 every month! Whereas uterus owners only have this magic pregnancy window for barely 3–5 days in a month. So, wouldn't it be more effective to target the millions of sperm? Well, yes of course! But is it easier? Umm . . . NO. And that's where the problem with male birth control lies. There are just so frikkin many sperm made all the frikkin time, that it is very hard to stop those little slippery swimmers. It's not because of a lack of people wanting to do that. It's because it's so hard! You'd still be quite fertile and produce millions of sperm even if your sperm count fell by 90 per cent! It is much easier to stop one egg being released every month than it is to stop hundreds of millions of sperm being produced every single day.

Now, birth control pills for women work in a very clever (and ironic) way—by mimicking a pregnancy. Once your body becomes pregnant, it will not release more eggs out into the wild for making Baby No. 2 while already pregnant, right? Instead, it will release some hormones that prevent the new egg from being released. Birth control pills contain these same hormones (that your body releases after ovulation) which make sure you don't immediately release more eggs. Now you start taking birth control pills at the beginning of your cycle, *before* ovulation has occurred. But from the very beginning of the cycle, these birth control pills maintain the hormonal bank balance that you would naturally have *after* ovulation. This makes your body think that ovulation has already happened, and your ovaries do not release more eggs. This is how 'anovulation' from birth control pills works, by mimicking a pregnancy.

If that was difficult to understand, think of it like this. Think of going to a restaurant and ordering food. Now, if you've ordered a massive chocolate cake to begin with, you won't go back and order a giant pizza *na*? (Okay fine, I know some of you will. No judgement. Just play along for my story, okay?). Instead, after eating the giant chocolate cake—think of this as ovulation—your body will release satisfaction chemicals inside you that make you feel full. This way you will not order the giant pizza. Now imagine there is a magical pill called NoMoreFood (think of this as birth control pills). NoMoreFood Pill contains the same chemicals your body naturally releases after eating cake (ovulation), which make sure you don't immediately order a new pizza (release new eggs). Now, you would take the NoMoreFood pill outside the restaurant, before you eat the cake. This way, from the very start of your restaurant visit, the NoMoreFood pill will maintain the satisfaction you would otherwise have after eating the cake. This makes your body think you are already full (have already ovulated), and you don't order the cake (anovulation), even though you never ate the cake to begin with. This is how birth control pills work.

Contrast this with sperm, which are produced fresh inside the testicles. At the start of puberty, your body makes a delicious testosterone milkshake, which is essential for the formation of these sperm. And once you start producing them, you never really stop. It's a 24/7 kinda situation. The only way to stop them would be to either completely shut down the testosterone milkshake production, or to block the road these sperm use to exit the body. We've actually already used that second option, since that's how a vasectomy works. Some scientists are also working on making a plug that you could inject inside the vas deferens, i.e., the tube that connects the testicles to the penis and helps transport sperm out, that could be dissolved with an injection if someone wanted to be fertile again. They're still going through trials for this as of 2022, so it may be a while before we see it in the market, if at all.

The problem with using the first option is that testosterone is a little bit essential for daily living. (As are estrogen and progesterone, but with birth control pills, we provide these hormones continuously, in amounts that our bodies naturally produce anyway during a part of our cycle. We don't stop them entirely. It's like giving you the same food every single day versus stopping food altogether.) Testosterone is essential for muscle and bone strength, among many other things. Stopping testosterone is not really an effective answer unless we could specifically stop testosterone locally only in the testicles. Luckily, for us, there is a group of doctors and scientists that are working on a drug that works locally on the testicles to reduce testosterone, and therefore sperm production. It's still in the works though.

So it's not that we aren't working on making alternative contraception options for men. We're working, and we're working very hard. Male contraception (other than condoms and surgery) is simply not at a stage where it can be considered safe and healthy by doctors and scientists. And I am not saying that there is no discrimination in medicine; there really is, and we are working on it, and will need to work on it for a very long time before it becomes even close to a level playing field. I'm saying that it's hard, and it will take some time for us to make a safe alternative that works as well. It's kinda like this: say you were to hear a really annoying tune on the TV. Would it not be easier to temporarily turn that TV off? Or would it make more sense to throw the whole TV out of the window to stop the song? Except it's not one TV, but 15 million of them.

24

Abortions

At the time of writing this chapter, there is a huge public debate in the US regarding the legality and morality of abortions. I will not get into any of that. My personal opinion means nothing, but I want you to know the facts so that you can make a decision for yourself if you are in the position of needing one. My job as a doctor is to empower you with knowledge that helps you make the best decision for your life and your body. I really don't care if you think abortion is right or wrong. No fun facts here, no history here. (Okay, maybe a little history. You know I love history.) This will be a straight-talking chapter where I will tell you in plain and simple language what an abortion is, how it's performed, what can be the side effects, and answer some common queries on abortions.

An abortion is a procedure with which you can end a pregnancy. An abortion is different from contraception; with contraceptives, we stop a pregnancy from happening all together. With abortions, we end a pregnancy that has already happened. Think of contraception like the friend zone. If you friendzone someone who asks you out, you will stop yourself from starting a relationship all together. Think of abortion like a break-up, it can help end a relationship that has already been established. Contraception can be of the regular type that you use routinely to stop a pregnancy, or it can be of the emergency type, which you use in an emergency (you can learn about this in the earlier chapter on contraception). *Contraception is not abortion.*

Abortion can sometimes happen on its own (when it's called a miscarriage or a spontaneous abortion) or it can happen with human intervention (when it's called an abortion). Abortion is a very common medical procedure, and people get abortions for all kinds of reasons. When they cannot access legal and safe abortions, people resort to dangerous, illegal, unsafe methods without medical supervision, which can lead to significant harm and even death. Globally, around 50–75 million abortions are performed every year although the number maybe different as some places do not report abortions due to the legality of the matter.

Abortions in India have been legal since 1971 though we have rules that define what is a legal abortion. Previously, abortions up to 20 weeks were allowed, but a new amendment in 2021 now permits abortions up to 24 weeks in special circumstances. Estimates say we see 6 million to 15 million abortions every year in India. There are various reasons under which you can get an abortion, such as:

- Any threat to the physical or mental health of the pregnant woman due to the pregnancy
- Risk to the health of the child
- If the pregnancy is caused due to sexual assault

-    If you used contraception, but it failed
-    Poor socioeconomic status

We've had various updates to this law in the past 51 years, which have made it more inclusive (but we can still do a lot more). You don't have to be legally married to have an abortion, and as long as you are over 18 years of age, you don't need permission from anyone else to have an abortion. Your consent is the only thing that matters. You are also not required to pay more if you are unmarried and having an abortion. In India, it's completely legal to *request* an abortion up to 20–24 weeks, as an adult.

There are two main kinds of abortions you could be offered: medical or surgical. Both procedures are extremely safe, effective, and do not impact your long-term fertility (if performed safely). The kind of abortion you get depends on the age of your pregnancy, your overall health, and what is preferable for you. You can calculate the age of your pregnancy by counting down from the first date of your last period. For example, if you had your last period on the 1st of April and today is the 1st of June, then you are eight weeks pregnant, as it has been eight weeks since you last had your period.

Medical Abortions

In India, we usually perform medical abortions in early pregnancy, up to 9 weeks. This is a simple, non-invasive, and cheaper method to abort using drugs. Almost 40 per cent of pregnancies worldwide are unplanned, so abortion pills can be very helpful. But please don't just buy the pills from a pharmacy and use them on your own. Not only is this illegal, but also if the pregnancy is in the wrong location, using abortion pills can cause life-threatening bleeding and complications. Please see a doctor before you choose to get an abortion, so they can estimate the age and location of your pregnancy and take care of your well-being, during and after the procedure.

We use two drugs for this: mifepristone (we'll call this the anti-Bournvita drug) and misoprostol (we'll call this the lemon drug). The process is started by using the anti-Bournvita drug, mifepristone. Every pregnancy needs nourishment, something like Bournvita for the embryo, to help it grow. Our body makes a natural embryo Bournvita in the form of progesterone that nourishes the pregnancy. Mifepristone, the anti-Bournvita drug, works by blocking the action of progesterone. Using our anti-Bournvita drug (mifepristone), we block the body's natural Bournvita (progesterone) and stop the growth of the embryo. Then, we add misoprostol (the lemon drug). Misoprostol does two things: (1) it works on the cervix, which is the exit point of your uterus, and makes it soft (so everything can exit the uterus easily) and (2) it causes contractions inside the uterus, so whatever is inside the uterus can easily be squeezed out, like juicing a lemon.

And so, the anti-Bournvita drug and the lemon drug work together to help remove a pregnancy that has already been established. Your doctor will perform an ultrasound to make sure that the pregnancy is inside the uterus (and not fixed outside the uterus, something called an ectopic pregnancy) and also take a detailed medical history to ensure you can safely use these pills. Some blood tests may also be done to ensure your safety. After this, the doctor will prescribe these pills to you, explain how to use them, and monitor your condition. Once you start with these pills, you will have period-like bleeding. There can be clots and painful cramps, which will be most intense in the first two days. Eventually, things will settle down in a week's time. It's basically like having a more painful period.

It sounds pretty chill, because it is a chill procedure (when used correctly). You want to make sure you're using these under medical supervision, or it can get complicated. For example, there are certain conditions in which you shouldn't be using abortion pills. If you have an IUD, or if you are on certain medications, or if you have a bleeding disorder or an allergy, or if the pregnancy is ectopic, i.e., it's fixed outside the uterus (yeah, that can happen!), we prefer using other methods of abortions, or you can have serious complications. Complications can include things like allergies, incomplete abortions, or excessive bleeding. These can even turn life-threatening, so doing it under the supervision of a doctor is the best and safest idea.

Also, it's totally illegal for the pharmacist to sell you these pills without a prescription. Like go-to-jail *waala* illegal.

Surgical Abortions

After nine weeks, abortions in India are performed surgically. This is a safe and effective operation which can be used to abort an unwanted pregnancy or help manage a miscarriage. You will be required to go to a doctor for this, as it's . . . umm . . . quite difficult to perform a surgery on yourself.

When you go to the doctor, they will do an ultrasound to calculate the age and location of your pregnancy, and then run some blood tests. They will do this to establish your health status and your safety for surgery. The hospital may ask you to come with someone else, as you will need physical and mental support, but this is not mandatory. Once your consent is taken, the ultrasound is done, and your blood reports look fine, your doctor will take you in for the procedure.

You'll be given a few medicines to help with the procedure. The doctor will give you the lemon drug (from the medical abortions) to make your cervix soft. This is important so that the surgeon can easily enter the uterus and help manage the pregnancy. This also helps because the cervix can serve as a natural opening into the body and we don't have to make any additional cuts. Then, they will give you some pain medicines so you are comfortable, and maybe also some anti-anxiety medicines. Finally, the doctors will give you some anaesthetic medicines to make you sleepy and make the experience pain-free. And then the procedure begins!

Your doctor will perform another ultrasound just to get a clear understanding of the inside situation. Then they will clean your vulva and vagina to ensure no infections happen and enter the cervix. Using a spoon-shaped instrument called a 'curette', the doctors will scrape out the inside lining (endometrium) and the pregnancy. Then, they might perform a repeat ultrasound to make sure everything is clean and clear, and that's it! It's barely a ten- to thirty-minute procedure. You might experience some bleeding after the procedure, but it won't be like a full period. And that's it! After some observation time, you'll be okay to go home. You'll be given some antibiotics to prevent any infections, and you'll be instructed to not insert anything into the vagina, such as tampons, menstrual cups, or a penis, for a few weeks.

Abortions are one of the safest medical procedures out there. The doctors will take good care of you. With that said, all medical procedures have some risks, and so do abortions. Infections, injuries, bleeding, allergies, or failure of surgery are some of the things that can go wrong. The doctor who is performing the surgery will know how to handle these complications.

Bus. Ho gaya. Kahaani khatam, paisa hazam.

FAQs

1. Is anyone else's consent required for you to have an abortion?
- Nope. As long as you are over 18 years of age, and are of 'sound mind', you only need your own consent. Not your parents', not your husband's, not your boyfriend's, not your girlfriend's, not your *dur waali taiji's*. Your consent is all that matters.
2. What if I am not 18?
- If you are under the age of 18, the consent of your parent or guardian is required. Since the age of consent in India is 18, any sex before the age of 18 counts as a statutory rape. So, pregnancies in people under the age of 18 are legally required to be reported to the police, and additional consent is needed.
3. What documents will be required?
- Your doctor will ask you for a government-issued ID, for record-keeping purposes and as a proof of age. This will

be kept confidential. The doctor may also ask after your past medical history and any conditions you might have.

4. Do I need to be married to have an abortion?
- Nope. Your marital status has nothing to do with getting an abortion.

5. Are there any long-term side effects?
- Abortion is an incredibly safe medical procedure. With that said, there are risks with everything. Sometimes, there are rare and serious complications that are beyond the control of your doctor. Sometimes, complications are not treated in time. Aside from these rare conditions, safe abortions do not affect your overall health. They don't make you infertile in the future. You can plan and have a baby in the future when you want. But please follow up with your doctor to get on some contraceptive plan after your abortion, so you can use a regular birth control method.

6. Other myths?
- Abortions don't cause breast cancer, infertility, or PCOS. Abortions don't make your uterus weak.

Human beings have been getting abortions or trying to perform abortions since time immemorial. Because of the lack of right knowledge, people have used dangerous techniques, from using poisonous plants to injuring themselves with knitting needles. Limiting access to abortion will not stop abortions, it will only increase unsafe abortions.

I hope you leave this chapter feeling empowered about your body and your rights.

Ohemgee! What's Wrong with Me?!

25

House of Horrors

Part I

For as long as human beings have been having sex, we have been getting STIs. STIs changed the world—syphilis *ko hi dekh lijiye*. And yet, just like sex and anything associated with it, STIs continue to be one of the most taboo subjects in the world. But for something that has had such a huge impact on history, be it syphilis in the 16th century or AIDS in the 21st century, why are we never educated about it? Estimates say that currently there are 1.1 billion (yes, billion) people in the world who have STIs other than HIV. It's very funny to me that the word 'stigma' starts with the letters STI, when STIs are so heavily stigmatized. Most of us have very little understanding of STIs, except that we make a few (insensitive) jokes about AIDS with friends. And so, after giving you this unnecessary long history lesson, I will give you some actual relevant information on STIs. I will start with syphilis but I promise I will not bore you with ancient syphilis.

Syphilis

Caused by: a bacteria called Treponema Pallidum.

Spread by: the vulva, vagina, penis, anus, or mouth touching a syphilis sore. Or from mom to baby (congenital syphilis).

Symptoms:
- There could be no symptoms at all.
- A round, painless sore on the genitals or mouth that lasts around three to six weeks. This will go away on its own in some time, but still needs treatment.
- If not treated at the sore stage, you could get rashes on the soles of your feet and your palms.
- There is body ache, sore throat, fever, and weight loss.
- Eventually can progress to blindness, paralysis, and nervous system damage, if not treated.

Detected by: a medical examination, a simple blood test, and a fluid sample taken from any ulcer or sore you might have.

Treated by: antibiotics.

Prevention: use condoms, dental dams, and get tested for STIs regularly.

HPV

If you've come here from my Instagram page, you may probably already know about HPV. If you haven't, don't worry, I'll still tell you all about it. HPV is considered the most common STI globally. HPV is a family of around 200 viruses that can cause sexual and non-sexual problems, and even cancer. HPV is so incredibly common that most people get HPV at some point in their lives with absolutely no symptoms or problems. In fact, if you've been sexually active, you've probably had HPV at some point in your life. If you have had more than three partners, your risk of getting HPV goes up six times. Most of the time, it's cleared by your immune system on its own. Sometimes it's not. But two types of HPV (16 and 18) are linked to a deadly cancer called cervical cancer, and other cancers of the genitals, mouth, and throat.

Caused by: a virus called Human Papillomavirus.

Spread by: skin-to-skin contact with the infected area. This can happen through touching the infected area and then touching other surfaces, and vaginal, anal, or oral sex.

Symptoms:
- Most people don't have any symptoms until it develops into something more serious
- Warts

Complications: various kinds of cancers.

Detected by: regular cervical smears during gynaecological examinations (get one every three years after you become sexually active).

Prevention: use condoms, dental dams, and get Pap smears regularly, and get the vaccines!

HPV vaccines protect against up to nine strains of HPV, including the cancer-causing ones. It's best to get the vaccine before you become sexually active, but you can still get it after becoming sexually active (because maybe you haven't been exposed to the cancer-causing strains). Getting the vaccine after getting infected with those particular strains won't do anything. Ideally, you get it between nine to thirteen years of age, but you can get it up to forty-five years of age. (You might see some Google search results showing that it's only up to the age of twenty-six, but that was data from before 2018. In 2018, it was approved for up to forty-five years.) Since September 2021, the vaccine is also available for and recommended to penis owners. In India, we have two kinds of vaccines available: Gardasil 4, which protects against four strains, and Gardasil 9, which protects against nine strains. As of late 2022, there is also a cheaper *swadesi* vaccine being developed, which will protect people from four strains. You can get whichever is easily available and fits your budget, since both vaccines protect from the cancer-causing strains.

Herpes

Herpes is like that charming fuckboi who promises he's different from other STIs (it's a virus, not a bacteria), but actually is just annoying, doesn't take no for an answer (symptoms can keep recurring, and the virus stays in your body for life), and causes you a lot of pain (like a lot). Just like there are fuckbois all around us, herpes is also very common.

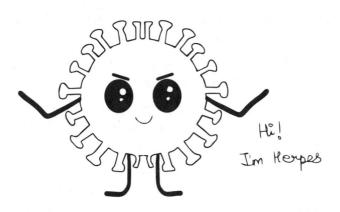

Hi!
I'm Herpes

Caused by: viruses called HSV1 and HSV2.

Spread by: skin-to-skin contact with the infected area. This can happen through kissing, vaginal sex, anal sex, or oral sex.

Symptoms:

- Painful blisters around your genitals, anus, or inner thighs
- Itching
- Pain with peeing if the sore is in the way of your urine
- Fever, chills, body ache

The first time you have sores after getting infected, it's called your first outbreak, and it lasts anywhere between two to four weeks. The herpes virus then stays in your body forever and can cause more outbreaks during times of stress. But it gets less painful over the years.

Complications: herpes in babies can be fatal, but adult herpes is not deadly and doesn't lead to any serious complications.

Detected by: a medical examination and a sample taken from the blister using a simple cotton earbud.

Treated by: well, it's not really treated since it basically stays with you forever. Pain relief, ice packs, and avoiding your trigger can be helpful in managing and preventing an episode.

Prevention: use condoms, dental dams, and get tested for STIs regularly. Herpes can also spread from non-sexual body parts so you can't really fully prevent it. But if you see your partner has herpes blisters, avoid sex with them during that time.

Chlamydia

Chlamydia is one of the most common STIs in the world, and *the* most common STI in India. It is also one of the most silent infections, as most people show no symptoms at all. And when the symptoms do turn up, it's often weeks after being infected. The most common symptom is increased discharge from the vagina or penis.

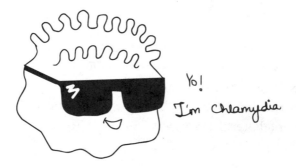

Yo! I'm Chlamydia

Caused by: a bacteria called Chlamydia Trachomatis.

Spread by: vaginal, anal, or oral sex. Or from mom to baby. Can also (rarely) spread by touching your eyes with hands that have infected fluid on them. So please wash your hands before you touch your eyes, especially your contact lenses!

Symptoms:
- There may be no symptoms at all. This is the most common symptom.
- Pain during sex or peeing
- Bleeding between periods
- Abnormal vaginal discharge
- Abnormal discharge from the penis
- Swollen testicles (*tatte sooj jaana* is a real medical thing, it turns out)
- Pain or itchiness around the butthole

Complications: pelvic inflammatory disease (PID), where the disease spreads in towards your uterus and Fallopian tubes. PID can cause long-term damage, and lead to infertility and an increased risk of ectopic pregnancies. In men, it can lead to inflammation of the prostate, and maybe even infertility.

Detected by: a medical examination, a simple urine test, and a sample taken from the urethra, vagina, cervix, anus, or tip of the penis using a simple cotton earbud.

Treated by: antibiotics.

Prevention: use condoms, dental dams, and get tested for STIs regularly.

Gonorrhoea

Another very common STI, commonly called 'the clap' (probably because French brothels were referred to as Le Clapier, and it was assumed that everyone got the clap from sex workers). Another theory is that one would 'clap' their penis between their hands to reduce the pain from the disease, which makes absolutely no sense to me. Like chlamydia, gonorrhoea also causes almost no symptoms at all. The most common symptoms are painful peeing, (what is often described as 'pissing razor blades') and discharge from the penis. This is where the name gonorrhoea comes from—gonos meaning seed aka semen, and orrhea meaning flow. So, it would literally be the flow of semen from the penis.

Caused by: a bacteria called Neisseria Gonorrhoea.

Spread by: vaginal, anal, or oral sex by contact with pre-cum, semen, or vaginal fluid. Or from mom to baby, which causes gonorrhoea in the baby's eyes. You can also get gonorrhoea in your throat from oral sex.

Symptoms:
-   There could be no symptoms at all. This is the most common symptom, especially for people with a vagina.
-   Pain during pooping or peeing
-   Bleeding between periods
-   Abnormal vaginal discharge
-   Abnormal discharge from the penis
-   Discharge from your butt
-   Swollen testicles

- Pain or itchiness around the butthole
- Sore throat

Complications: PID, where the disease spreads in towards your uterus and Fallopian tubes. PID can cause long-term damage, and lead to infertility and an increased risk of ectopic pregnancies. In men, it can lead to inflammation of the prostate, and maybe even infertility.

Detected by: a medical examination, a simple urine test, and a sample taken from the urethra, vagina, cervix, anus, or tip of the penis using a simple cotton earbud.

Treated by: antibiotics.

Prevention: use condoms, dental dams, and get tested for STIs regularly.

There are a few more STIs, but I took you through a highlight reel to show you two main things: 1) STIs often have no symptoms, so don't wait for a problem to get tested. Get regular STI tests to keep yourself and your partner safe. 2) The prevention for all STIs is the same: use condoms and dental dams for ANY kind of sex: vaginal, anal, or oral. These two simple things cover everything you need to know about STIs (sorry for wasting your time by making you read all of that).

* * *

We have historically associated a lot of shame with STIs because they were thought to be a punishment from God, and sex was considered immoral if it was done for anything other than making babies. But we now know both of these things are not true, and STIs have always been supremely widespread. They're as common as the common cold, and you wouldn't judge anyone for having a cold, would you? Extend that same courtesy to yourself and your partner when it comes to sex and sexual health. There has been a huge rise in the number of STI cases in the world in the past few years, and more and more are becoming antibiotic-resistant. Use simple safe-sex practices to prevent their further spread. Ideally, you should be having an STI test every year that you are sexually active, and a new test before you get a new partner. This way, you stay safe, they stay safe, and we all live healthily ever after. (Happily ever after is a myth in this economy.)

26

House of Horrors

Part 2

I feel like we haven't done a quiz in a while, so let's go!

Q1. STIs are the only problems you can have in your genitals.
   A) Yeah, duh
   B) Dude, no. There's so many more
   C) I have no idea

Q2. You can't have more than one STI at the same time.
   A) Nah, you can have a whole party in your genitals!
   B) Yeah, only one infection happens at a time
   C) Only people with penises can have multiple STIs

Q3. It's normal for sex to hurt.
   A) Yeah, but only for the first time
   B) Yes, sex is usually painful for women
   C) Nope, sex is not supposed to hurt

Q4. Are there any contraceptives that protect you from STIs?
   A) Yeah, condoms, and IUDs
   B) Yeah, condoms only

   C) Nope, we need to take medicines to protect us
      from STIs

Answer key 1B, 2A, 3C, 4B

I'm hoping that you've scored 4/4 on this quiz, because
you've already read a whole book's worth of information
about the wonderful adventures of humans and sex. You've
also learnt a bunch of animal sex facts, actually. But we still
have some more genitals problems to learn about, so let's do
a House of Horrors Part 2 to learn about vulva- and vagina-
specific issues.

   (If you do experience any of these symptoms, please see
a doctor so you can get an accurate diagnosis and the right
treatment.)

Bumps and Boils

So, you shaved and now your vulva is covered in these weird
bumps. These bumps are called ingrown hairs and they're
like air bubbles trapped under a new sheet of tempered glass
on your phone. Normally, after hair removal, your hairs are
supposed to grow out of the follicles, straight up and out.
But sometimes, they get trapped under the skin, creating
a bump. It usually looks like a small pimple, having a little
bit of pus in it, and may be slightly tender to the touch.
Sometimes, they can get infected and become extremely
tender and cause a lot of pain.

   A simple way to avoid these ingrown hairs is to always
shave in the direction of the hair growth. Do not go against

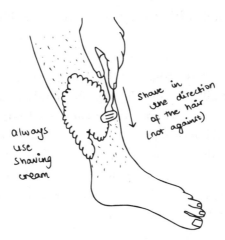

always
use
shaving
cream

Shave in
the direction
of the hair
(not against)

the grain, as it increases your chances of getting ingrown hair. Always shave in the shower, after using some warm water to soften up the hair. Using a sharp new blade and some shaving cream every time you shave is also helpful. But, if you repeatedly get infected boils, it might be a good idea to see your doctor.

Bacterial Vaginosis

Remember our good friends the lactobacilli? The nice bacteria that live inside the vagina and protect it, preventing other microbes from living in your vagina apartment? Well, in bacterial vaginosis (BV), there is a reduced amount of these good lactobacilli, and an overgrowth of other harmful microorganisms. This bacterial overgrowth makes your body say 'vagin? No sis!' (Wow! that was a terrible joke even by my standards) and leads to a thin, greyish, smelly discharge from your vagina. It's usually described as smelling 'fishy' or 'ammonia' like.

Bacterial vaginosis can be caused due to a number of reasons, the most common being douching. When you douche, you kill our good lactobacili friends who cannot do their job of protecting you any longer. This leads to bacterial overgrowth. BV is seen more in sexually active women; having a new or multiple partners increases your risk of getting bacterial vaginosis. Additionally, having BV increases your risk of getting other STIs. Using condoms protects you from this fishy-smelling vaginal discharge and interestingly, being on the birth control pill also reduces your risk. Basically, use condoms, don't douche, and let your vagina do its thing. It'll take care of itself.

Fungal Infections

Have you ever had an intensely itchy itch in your groin? The kind you could scratch forever but that still wouldn't go away, but only made your skin raw? Like wake you up in the middle of the night just to *khujao* like a madman? You probably have a fungal infection!

It can cause itching, burning, a discharge that looks like curd (dahi), penis/vulva and vagina swelling, and pain with sex. Usually, your good lactobacilli prevent this fungus, candida, from over-growing, but certain conditions can cause candida overgrowth: long-term antibiotic use, pregnancy, uncontrolled diabetes, or a weakened immune system.

Treatment involves basic anti-fungal medication given by your doctor and avoiding clothing that traps moisture.

Vaginismus

Sometimes your vagina can get inspired by a Venus flytrap and decide to shut the doors immediately when something comes close to entering it. Vaginismus is the involuntary (not under your control) clamping down of your vaginal muscles. This can happen with any penetration such as inserting a tampon or a medical device or inserting a penis or it can happen only on certain occasions. There can be several underlying reasons—shame at the idea of sex, infection, injury, or a history of sexual assault—and requires a multi-disciplinary treatment from a gynaecologist, a psychiatrist, and a pelvic floor therapist.

Bartholin Gland Cyst

There are two small glands situated near the opening of the vagina. They are called Bartholin's glands and they help produce lubrication for the vagina. Sometimes, the outlet of this duct can get blocked, like a traffic jam, and the pent-up fluids can cause the gland sac to become bigger. If infected, this becomes a round lump near the vaginal opening that is super tender, painful, and hot. Although we don't know what causes them, your gynaecologist can help you fix it if you have this condition.

Conclusion

This is not a book about sex.

This is a book about learning about your body and hopefully falling in love with it somewhere along the way. This is a book about unlearning the shame that's instilled in us from the very moment we are born. This is a book about understanding how things work, how your parts fit together. This is a book about empowering you with the right facts to make informed decisions about your health.

I don't like long goodbyes, so I will keep this short. I hope this book was helpful for you; it certainly was for me. I hope you learnt something about your body, your genitals, the culture of shame, your brain, intimacy, medicine, history, or whatever else you found useful in here. If not, I hope it at least made you laugh.

And that's the feeling I hope you will carry with yourself from here.

Byeeeeeeeeeeeee!

PS: There is nothing wrong with your body and you look beautiful the way you are. Don't let those evil illogical beauty standards win. Now byeeeee!

PPS: Vulva, not vagina!

Acknowledgements

This is the first chapter of my book that I wrote because it's seriously crazy that I am writing a book. I mean, really?! When did I become cool? And then I realized that I'm not actually cool, just surrounded by really really cool people who have rubbed off on me a little bit. So, let's thank all those cool people.

The coolness runs in the family, so I must start with thanking my family—mum, Bau, thank you for raising me up in such a chill environment, accepting my (many many) fuck-ups, and teaching me what sex-positive doctors are before I knew what sex-positive doctors are. You guys are the gods of cool. Bhaiya, thank you for teaching me how not to be a doormat, that being a nerd is really cool, and the importance of the Oxford comma. My life (and writing) would be nowhere without it. Yash, thank you for talking me out of anxiety spells when I had too many caffeine bars, even though I know coffee makes me anxious. My wonderful Chaturvedi *pariwar*, you have encouraged and inspired me in ways you will never know. Lyla (the OG), Coco, Coffee, and Samosa, your tail wags and barks have not just made me happier, but also inspired me to be a better human being (yes, I have a section thanking my dogs over the years, they are seriously very important). Samosa, thank you for waking me up at the ass crack of dawn everyday (for you to poop), for always sharing your food with me, and for keeping my feet warm while I write.

Anamika Aunty and Jaivardhan Uncle, thank you for existing, and encouraging me to give up my dreams of writing (lolol, joke's on you) and go to medical school. We probably wouldn't be here without it. Late Ravindra Tauji and Mamta Taiji, it was impossible not to want to become a writer, growing up under your literary genius—you have shaped my childhood, my dreams, and aspirations. Chhaya Aunty and Paritosh Uncle, you inspired me to keep pushing and working hard ever since I have known you. My dear little family, thank you for believing in me and loving me and teaching me so much.

Could not have done this without Srishti, Caro, Sarvari, Ankit, Shazia, Jayati, Isha, Liam, Chitra, Shambhavi, Pratha, Surbhi, and Somesh. Y'all have picked me up off the floor across various points in my life and told me to get my shit together, which has been pretty damn effective. You guys are the real pillars of my life and you know it. Thanks to my umbilical cord in Allahabad, Raghav and Anand Chachu for . . . just keeping shit together at home all the time. Roshni, my poshest Posh, thank you for getting Bhaiya off my back and always commenting hearts on my Instagram posts. Romika, thank you for saving my ass more times than I can count, legally and otherwise. Kushagra, thank you for sitting with me and drawing every single pubic hair over beers, at the very last moment for the illustrations!

Big thanks to Prahaar (Ajitabh, Kushal, Shreya, Vipul, Deepa, Vincent, Shivani, and Shaeba) for ENDLESSLY making fun of me and providing a lot of the jokes in this book; to my OxHoes (Meher, Shezae, and Maryam) and my nerd mini universe at Oxford (Gabi, Priyav, Deepanshu, Alistair, Peter, and Thao) for the constant entertainment, encouragement, and way too many wine and cheese nights; my lawyer gang (Suyukti, Dawar, Lalla, Chikki Dada, Shuklaji, Shivi, Himadri, Batra, Chhotu, Khanna-Khanni, Vishakha, William) for the endless laughter, drunken nights, and an opportunity to let my hair down during rather manic workdays; my piddi party at Ansals (Shubhankar, Varun, Shringar, Anand, and Chirag) for all the badminton games and support when Cuterus started, and my Instagram family (Nandini Didi, Anubha, Manas, Kushagra, Siddhant, Chirag, and Nadine) for the memes, love, and other drugs (JK JK JK). Thank you to Ami Patel, my therapist, for holding my life together through this crazy year. Thanks to Siddharth, for that wonderful night drinking Guinness at the Wetherspoons on George Street when I first told anyone in the world that I want to grow up and educate the world on sex.

Thanks to my angel manager, Anika, for making my life run effectively in the background while I buried myself in the writing process. Omkar Chincholkar and team, plus my PureYoga Texas crew are credited with forcing me to move my butt while I wrote. Big thank you to Bonobo and Four Tet for fantastic writing music, the University of Texas at Austin for fantastic writing environments, and CommonDesk Austin (especially the happy hours with Dalton, Marie, and Brooke) for channelling both of these and actually making me write.

Thank you to my smol kyootoo Instagram community for being there, offering valuable feedback on my content, and being so so full of love and support. You guys probably have no idea how dramatically you have changed my life and I could not be more thankful if I tried.

Most importantly, thank you to my editor and all-round champ human being, Shreya, for offering me this book deal, without which we wouldn't be here, and Tarini for taking over when Shreya abandoned me (sad reaccs only). Oh, and also believing in me and correcting my awful spellings and making this book kickass. (Yes, I'm calling my own book kickass and I know Shreya and Tarini agree. This is our baby.) This book would be nowhere without Binita, who made me realize how truly awful my grammar and spelling are, and politely fixed it all. Huge thanks to Ashish Langade from Three Little Words photography for driving down all the way from Pune to click my cover image and general tomfoolery through the day.

I am 100 per cent sure I have missed many names even though I have read and reread this about four thousand times, so I am sorry, and you know you have impacted my life in huge ways and I'm a shithead for forgetting to credit you. I will probably credit you in a gifted book with an extra note on the front page so please watch out for that.

Okay, I love you, thanks bye.